How to Lose Weight Without Dieting or Exercise.

Over 250 Ways.

Learn About Foods that Burn Fat, Weight Loss Diets, Weight Loss Tips, Weight Loss Foods, and How to Lose Belly Fat

By Dr. Ernesto Martinez

www.AttaBoyCowboy.com

Also by Ernesto Martinez

*How to Travel the World and Live with No
Regrets.
Learn How to Travel for Free, Find Cheap Places
to Travel, and Discover Life-Changing Travel
Destinations.*

*How to Boost Your Credit Score Range and Make
Money with Credit Cards.
How to Repair Your Credit with Credit Repair
Strategies.*

*How to Become Rich and Successful: Creative
Ways to Make Money with a Side Hustle
How to Become a Millionaire: Learn the Best
Passive Income Ideas*

*How to Heal Broken Bones Faster. Bone Fracture
Healing Tips.
Learn About Bone Fracture Healing Foods, Types
of Bone Fractures, and the Five Stages of Bone
Healing.*

*How to Become Rich and Successful. The Secret
of Success and the Habits of Successful People.
Entrepreneurship and Developing Entrepreneur
Characteristics*

How to Lose Weight Without Dieting or Exercise. Over 250 Ways.

Learn About Foods that Burn Fat, Weight Loss Diets, Weight Loss Tips, Weight Loss Foods, and How to Lose Belly Fat

DEDICATION

The family is one of nature's treasures. Love is the cement that binds us together, brings harmony and reduces friction. Thank you all for sharing this beautiful life with me.

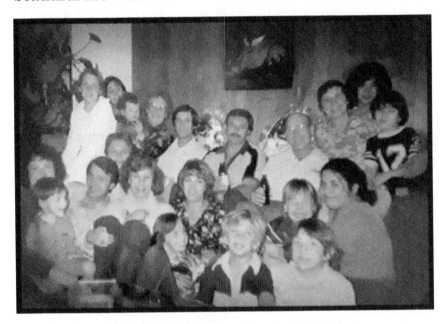

Table of Contents

Introduction

On 07/24/2020, I took a trip to Puerto Rico. Even though I followed every precaution recommended by the Centers for Disease Control (CDC), I caught Covid-19 by not remembering to use a paper towel to grab the bathroom handle on my way out of the bathroom on the plane. After three days, I started feeling headaches, dizziness, and fevers. On 08/05/2020, I tested positive for Covid-19. I started my near-death experience by fighting off Coronavirus for seven weeks and another two months afterward as a "long hauler," fighting off the long term effects of shortness of breath, lung scarring, and debility. Fortunately, I recovered most of my function to be faced with lockdowns and a new normal of extremely reduced physical activity. I no longer could go swimming in the public pool, workout at the gym, hike trails, and beaches have been closed off and on, and many of the places and friends I use to visit are no longer open to having guests due to the pandemic. I continued seeing patients and noticed a common occurrence as many of them gained weight, along with friends, family, and co-workers I would see through Zoom meetings. The new norm of weight gain became to be known as the "Quarantine 15".

Stress is a powerful appetite stimulant, but it does not reduce it. Self-isolation and sheltering in place during the COVID-19 pandemic is causing a 15-pound weight gain known as the "Quarantine 15." Although the average is around 8 pounds, the pandemic fueled weight gain is being compared to the "Freshman 15".

Research shows that the severity of stress that someone is exposed to can influence overall food intake and result in either under or overeating. Chronic stress feeds a greater preference for energy and nutrient dense foods, usually high sugar and fat foods. Other animal species have also been shown to gorge on sugar ladened foods over protein when under stress. Sugary foods are a potent energy source to feed an energized body in fight or flight mode quickly.

Many animals, like humans, often feed stress instead of managing it, leading to weight gain.

The Stress-Eating Cycle

When we're scared or worried, we're more likely to seek out carbs, sugars, and fats for a quick energy boost, such as increasing cravings for chocolate, pizza, and potato chips during the coronavirus quarantine. Comfort foods remind us of better times and act as natural tranquilizers that calm us down in times of danger.

However, a short term de-stressor can cause long term problems. Comfort eating can trap you into hard-to-break eating cycles that increase stress levels and health problems, such as heart disease, obesity, and diabetes, as well as emotional issues, such as anxiety and depression.

When stressed, the brain signals the stress hormones cortisol and adrenaline to be pumped into your bloodstream. This sequence also triggers glucose release from your liver and muscles, causing an energy spike and preparing you to defend yourself.

After a stressful experience, glucose levels must be replenished. So the more glucose we release during a stress reaction, the hungrier we'll be after the stressor. That increases our cravings for fats and sweets to replenish cortisol. The higher the stress, the larger the amounts of cortisol released, and the greater the cravings for foods high in salt, fat, and sugar, resulting in stress eating. The overconsumption of sugars and fats causes weight gain, fat storage, damage to our health, and creating the stress-eating cycle.

Breaking the Cycle

Maintaining an unhealthy diet will cause chronically elevated cortisol levels keeping you in a constant state of fight or flight. Our bodies are not meant to be in a chronic state of stress nor to use food for comfort. To break the stress cycle, we can engage in stress-reducing activities, such as yoga, physical exercise, and meditation. Coupling the activity with some of the over 250 healthy strategies explained here will give you healthier ways of managing unpredictable times, like the pandemic, and improving your overall health through lifestyle redesign.

Over 250 Ways to Lose Weight Without Exercise

A. Behaviors That Help You Lose Weight

1. Quench Food

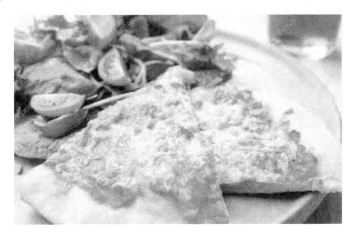

W hen I was studying nutrition at California State University Los Angeles (CSULA), I had a professor named Dr. Tam, Ph.D. who used to say we need to "quench foods." He taught us that it was o.k. to have cheat meals but to help quench some of the damage caused by the unhealthy meal. For example, if you like french fries and you order a side of fries, then eat a salad with it to counteract the damage caused by the fries. You don't have to give up your favorite foods completely. You should reduce the frequency of eating them and add something to the meal to reduce the total calories for the meal. If you eat a brownie, then eat an apple with it to increase the fiber intake, reduce overall calories, and add some nutrients. This simple strategy has been beneficial for me in managing my weight and the weight of my patients.

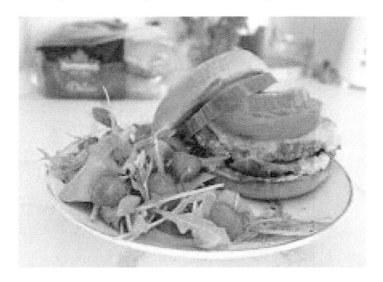

Think of a tea kettle; just as the water starts boiling it has to blow off some steam, otherwise, the steam would build up inside the pot and blow up. By allowing some steam to escape occasionally, the water can continue to boil as it reaches your desired temperature. Weight loss is the same in that you have to be forgiving and to redesign your eating habits to achieve your long term goals. Research shows that resisting food can cause your body to crave that food even more. Avoiding cookies or burgers wires your brain to view forbidden foods as rewards, making you crave foods that you have easy access to, so it's best to take a break if you need to and indulge every once in a while.

Weight loss can be difficult and frustrating; part of the solution is to be understanding and consider a lifestyle redesign. Including an imperfect diet as part of the plan will help you avoid the guilt and shame associated with perceived failure. When you eat that donut or bacon double cheeseburger, learn to accept cravings as part of life and to deal with the consequences in a standardized matter such as quenching. You'll have over 250 strategies to use to offset the meals that will be necessary on occasion to prevent binging.

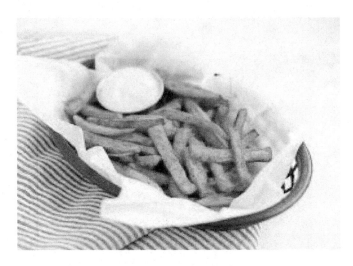

Crispy baked or air fried sweet potato fries

2. Don't Let Yourself Get Too Hungry

If you're too hungry, your gut will signal the reward system in your brain, so you start craving the worst foods first. Respond to feelings of hunger with healthy snacks to help keep these feelings and hormones in check.

However, if you eat too little, your brain will not signal the release of hormones that help you feel satiety. Therefore you'll continue to feel hungry. Smaller meals do not cause enough hormonal response to turn off hunger. You'll still be hungry and end up eating more than you should.

While overeating food is the most prominent cause of weight gain, eating too little can be one of the easiest ways to fail at weight loss. Your body has an instinct to protect itself. When you don't eat enough food and nutrients, your body will automatically go into starvation mode when deprived of such nutrition, causing the metabolism to slow down and the body to store any food eaten as fat. As a result, it will become much more difficult for you to lose weight.

3. Smell Your Food

Eighty percent of the flavors we taste come from what

we smell, which is why foods lose their flavor when we have a stuffy nose.

Smelling fresh-baked donuts can trigger you to start craving donuts, but it can also help you satisfy the urge to eat one. Studies show that participants exposed to an aroma will have a stronger desire for that food in the first 30 seconds, but after two minutes, they'll habituate and no longer crave the food. Many of the participants started craving fruit instead.

When you smell a fragrant but unhealthy food, pathways in your brain become excited by the new scent. As your senses habituate to the aroma, the neurons in your brain stop firing with the same frequency. Similar to the first bite of something delicious being the best, your senses get used to the taste and smell, and it doesn't elicit a strong response.

All five of our senses use habituation to adapt to our environment. Habituation is used by your body to calm itself. Another example would be walking into a room with a noticeably pungent odor. But, after being in the place long enough, the smell gradually becomes less noticeable. By the time you exit the room, the scent may not register at all.

You can use habituation to help yourself lose weight by narrowing down food options you eat every day, so you aren't tempting your nose and taste buds with too many novel stimuli. People eat more when exposed to more food options. That's why buffets cause you to gain weight because it's hard to habituate when there are various new foods to try.

Food aromas can also affect you in a good or bad way psychologically by triggering memories associated with certain foods. For example, smelling fresh-baked pumpkin pie could bring back memories of childhood and a parent who baked delicious comfort foods that made you feel safe. The craving you have for a piece of pumpkin pie isn't real hunger but the need to feel comforted.

That's what distinguishes cravings from real hunger. When it's true hunger, you'll eat anything. In contrast, desires are for specific foods, often unhealthy ones, and often triggered by stress. One of the best ways to distinguish a craving from real hunger is to ask yourself if you'd be satisfied with an apple. If the answer is yes, you're hungry. But, if only a chocolate brownie or chocolate chip cookie will suffice, it's a craving.

Scents of certain foods like extra-virgin olive oil suppress cravings and help you feel fuller. Smelling dark chocolate can lower levels of the appetite hormone ghrelin and suppress your appetite. The aroma of fresh green apples, bananas, and pears can help curb appetite and lessen cravings for sugary desserts. Scented lotion can also help decrease your desire to eat.

When I used to eat meat, fried fish, and chicken were my favorite dishes. When I walk into a dinner party and smell a meat dish that triggers a craving, I'll grab a leftover piece and smell it for a minute or until it no longer smells delicious or makes my mouth water. This strategy has helped me erase urges for meat dishes whenever they arise and has kept me a vegetarian for over sixteen years.

4. Use Post-it Notes

Leaving yourself Post-it messages helps reprogram your subconscious mind and help you stay focused on goals. Leaving yourself motivational messages urging you to eat healthily can help keep you focused on eating right and reaching your weight loss goals.

The three steps to being successful with Post-it notes:

• Make a list of your top three goals, such as buying a house, traveling to Los Angeles, or losing weight.

• Break down each goal into manageable steps. Every step needs to be something you can accomplish in a reasonable amount of time each day in no more than 20 minutes. For example, if your goal is to fit into a new dress, some small steps may include joining a gym, getting rid of processed food in your fridge, or learning to cook a fresh, healthy meal.

• Place your motivational messages in places where you're sure to see them throughout the day. Some key areas can include the bathroom mirror, fridge, car radio, or computer screen at work. When you feel like your motivation is lagging, work on a few minor steps towards one of your goals. By starting small, you'll soon be crossing off both major and minor goals that increase your quality of life. By starting, you'll be on your way to accomplishing your goals, no matter how small the steps are.

5. Not Eating After You Exercise

After exercise you may not feel hungry, so you don't eat. The problem is that workouts deplete muscle stores, and eating the right mix of nutrients within an hour after you finish helps them recover, which is essential for increasing lean muscle mass. After you exercise, eat a snack made up of 10 to 15 grams of protein and 15 grams of carbs.

6. Hide Unhealthy Foods

Avoid the see-food diet, when you see food and immediately eat it. Think about when you go to the grocery store, and you see all the candy bars by the checkout. You're stuck standing in line staring at the candies, and you start thinking about eating them, even though you'd probably like to avoid them. Candies are placed in this location to trigger impulse buying and eating of the store's most profitable junk food. Keeping unhealthy foods visible can trigger "visual hunger," an evolutionary trait that increases levels of hunger hormones when we see food. You want to remove the same type of temptation in your home and instead keep a bowl of fruit in its place.

Store unhealthy foods out of sight, in dark containers, in cabinets, pantries, or your desk, so you don't notice them when you're hungry. Keep healthy foods visible on your countertops, desktop, front, and center in your fridge, and plain sight. Strategically storing your food, will help support healthy eating and weight loss.

7. Don't Shame Yourself

Some people think that criticizing and harassing themselves or others may help them lose weight. However, instead of motivating people, it makes people feel bad about themselves, causing them to eat more and gain more weight. Stigma and discrimination against overweight people cause significant psychological harm and make the problem worse. People who experience weight discrimination were 6.67 times more likely to become obese, and 3.2 times more likely to remain obese.

Weight discrimination can cause depression, eating disorders, reduced self-esteem, and an increased risk of various other mental and physical problems. Being obese increases your risk of suicide by 21 times. Being kinder to yourself and others will help people lose weight faster.

8. Serve Meals in Multiple Small Portions

Instead of serving all of your food onto one plate, split your meal onto multiple plates. Using multiple plates will make it seem like you are eating much more than you really are, so you get fuller faster. This method is very helpful if you're in a buffet. Studies have shown that when the same amount of food is divided up onto multiple plates, the person gets full faster eating on multiple plates versus eating the same amount of food on one plate.

9. Serve Yourself

According to researchers at the University of Southern California (USC), the less physically involved we are in serving ourselves food, the more easily we deny responsibility for unhealthy eating or large portions.

Serving yourself is self-incriminating, so you're more likely to ask yourself with every spoon or scoop full if you need more and if you're willing to pay the consequences for indulging in something unhealthy. When someone else serves your plate, or you grab a pre-packaged meal, it's easier to overeat because you can blame someone else, and therefore, don't have to feel responsible for eating that extra dessert or portion.

10.   Serve Yourself Before You Sit

Family dinners are excellent, but make sure to serve yourself before sitting at the table. When food is right in front of you at the dinner table, and within reach, it's harder to turn it away. When you line up food buffet-style on the countertop, instead of laying out each dish on the dining room table, it makes people think twice before getting up to serve themselves again.

11.   Listen to Classical Music

Soft lighting and music can help you eat less and help you enjoy your food more. Listening to soft music such as Mozart can help improve metabolism, food digestion, overall health, and help you lose weight. Listening to rock or pop music can cause you to eat at a faster pace. When you eat while listening to pop or rock music, you automatically start eating faster and often overeat.

12.   Choose Quality over Quantity

Research shows that restrained eaters end up consuming more of the unhealthy foods they're trying to avoid. Restrained eaters experience more food cravings and are more likely to overeat the foods they crave. Give in to your desires on occasion, but try choosing a treat that also packs a nutritional punch, such as dark chocolate with fresh fruit.

13.   Avoid Frequency Eating

You've probably heard the advice that eating small meals throughout the day is the best way to speed up your metabolism and help you lose weight.

However, research has shown zero benefits to eating multiple meals a day to speed up your metabolism or promote weight loss. Research has shown that eating six meals a day made people want to eat more and effectively gain weight. The more frequently people eat, the higher their total calorie intake tends to be for the day.

14. Beware of Relationship Pounds

The average person gains 17 pounds within the first year of dating and 36 pounds since meeting their partner. After finding a partner, three-quarters of people felt less pressure to look their best and end up gaining weight.

People in relationships spend more time eating together, watching TV, drinking alcohol, and even if they ate healthier food, their portions tend to be larger. Couples also experience decreased physical activity and a decline in weight maintenance to attract an intimate partner.

Breakups had the opposite effect and helped facilitate weight loss. Other than a breakup, the key is to develop healthy habits together, such as working out, going for walks, or setting fitness goals together.

15. Be Affectionate

Studies show that kissing, hugging, snuggling, and holding hands can increase levels of the feel-good hormone, oxytocin. It can boost overall health, help you lose weight, lower blood pressure, fight off sickness, and decrease appetite.

16. Hang Out with More Females

Men are more likely to overeat and over drink when hanging out with other men. Even if men aren't thinking about it, eating more or pounding a few extra beers, is a demonstration of virility and strength. So eat and drink before meeting up with friends, see your guy friends one at a time, or go on a date with a girlfriend. Women on the other hand tend to eat less when they're with their girlfriends.

17. Avoid Decision Fatigue

Decision fatigue is the deteriorating quality of decisions made by a person after a long session of decision making. Decision fatigue can cause people to make poor eating choices, leading to weight gain. Meal prepping for the week can help prevent making poor eating decisions due to decision fatigue. People who are good at making decisions called "skill discretion" can get things done themselves and tend to have lower BMI. On the other hand, people who make several decisions for others can experience decision fatigue and make poor choices, such as ordering an extra serving of dessert.

18. Intermittent Fasting

Intermittent fasting, also known as intermittent energy restriction, is cycling between voluntary fasting and non-fasting over a given period.

Three methods of intermittent fasting are time-restricted eating, alternate-day fasting, and periodic fasting:

• Time-restricted eating means you only eat for a certain number of hours each day. Also known as skipping a meal and the 16:8 diet, 16 fasting hours cycled by eight non-fasting hours, for example eating from 10 am to 6 pm. The most common type of intermittent fasting practiced.

• Alternate-day fasting is alternating between a 24-hour fast when the person eats less than 25% of usual caloric needs, followed by a 24-hour non-fasting period. It is the most rigorous form of intermittent fasting because there are more days of fasting per week.

There are three subtypes:

❏ Complete alternate-day fasting, also known as total intermittent energy restriction, where you eat nothing on fast days.

❑ Modified alternate-day fasting, also known as partial, intermittent energy restriction, where you eat up to 25% of your daily caloric needs on fasting days instead of complete fasting.

❑ Periodic fasting, whole-day fasting, or the 5:2 diet; only eat 500-600 or about 25% of regular daily caloric intake on two days of the week but eat your typical food the other five days.

As long as you don't overeat, outside of fasting periods, fasting is beneficial for weight loss. The main reason that intermittent fasting can work, is that you'll have much fewer opportunities to eat, which can be a beneficial long-term behavioral change. In addition, the body stores calories in the form of body fat, and burns those calories whenever we don't eat.

Here are some of the hormones that change when you fast:

❑ Human growth hormone (HGH): During fasting, HGH increases as much as 5-fold. HGH, produced by the pituitary gland, decreases fat, and increases body fluids, muscle and bone growth, sugar, and fat metabolism.

❑ Insulin: Insulin increases when we eat and decreases when we don't. Lower levels of insulin facilitate fat burning.

❑ Norepinephrine (noradrenaline): Norepinephrine is sent by the central nervous system to break down fat cells into free fatty acids that can be burned for energy, which causes a boost in metabolism.

Fasting is more effective at fat burning than eating 5-6 meals a day. On average, intermittent fasters lost about 0.55 pounds (0.25 kg) per week, and alternate-day "fasters" lost 1.65 pounds (0.75 kg) per week.

Intermittent fasting is an easy way to restrict calories without consciously trying to eat less. It also allows you to build muscle while fasting, lose weight, reduce belly fat, and extend lifespan. One of the worst side effects of most diets is that you lose up to 25% of your muscle along with body fat.

To magnify the effects of intermittent fasting, you still need to eat healthy and decrease caloric intake. For extra weight loss, eat smaller meals to boost your metabolism within your fasting time. Some researchers recommend keeping your snacks to 100-200 calories and small meals to 300-400 calories.

19.   Juice Fasting can Help Balance Hormones

Your overall health will depend on your body's homeostasis. Eating an unhealthy diet, poor nutrition, stress, illness, genetics, or environmental factors, can cause hormonal imbalance in the body. Depending on the magnitude of the imbalance, you may experience weight gain, fatigue, and dysfunction in just about any one of your body systems.

Juicing for 3-30 days can help you reset your hormones, improve blood sugar control, promote weight loss, and get your health back on track. Juicing removes the fiber and allows your body to access large amounts of highly concentrated and absorbable nutrients. The large quantities of micronutrient minerals, vitamins, enzymes, and phytonutrients support anti-inflammatory actions and healthy cellular function in the hormonal glands and cells.

Juicing will also help detox and heal your liver. The liver is responsible for regulating, excreting, and breaking down our hormones for elimination via the kidneys and bowels. Juices and plant-based nutrients can stimulate the growth of healthy liver cells, thus improving function. Use a rainbow of mostly vegetables and some fruits in your juices to support and balance your hormone levels.

20.   Eating Breakfast

The word "breakfast" comes from the phrase "breaking

the fast." We fast while we sleep, and what we eat when we break that fast is central to rapid weight loss. Keep in mind that there is no set time for breakfast, and eating breakfast can be combined with intermittent fasting. So, you may eat your breakfast at 10:00 am, rather than 7:00 am, but you're still breaking the fast and maintaining your fast.

Eating breakfast is essential to boosting your metabolic rate throughout the rest of the day. However, it is crucial to avoid eating only carbohydrates, such as a bagel or cereal for breakfast. Add at least 29 grams of protein to your breakfast to keep you satiated longer. It takes more energy to digest protein than carbs, and it promotes muscle mass.

21. Eat a Larger Breakfast and Smaller Dinner

Your most substantial meal of the day should be your first meal of the day. Eating a big breakfast will help you burn twice as many calories for the rest of the day when compared to those who eat a more substantial dinner. If you eat a low-calorie breakfast, you're more likely to snack throughout the day. Also, eating a smaller breakfast causes you to eat larger meals at dinner, which results in weight gain. A large dinner also has adverse effects on glucose tolerance, which affects diabetic patients trying to avoid a spike in blood glucose. Therefore, a large breakfast is preferred over a large dinner to reduce the risk of metabolic diseases.

Measuring your diet-induced thermogenesis (DIT), will tell you how well your body metabolizes food, rate your hunger, measure blood glucose levels, and cravings for sweets. After a morning meal, your DIT increases by 2.5 higher when compared to after dinner. Besides, eating a high-calorie breakfast was linked to lower hunger, sweet cravings, lower insulin, and blood glucose levels throughout the day compared with after dinner.

22. Turn Down the Temperature in Your Home

Humans are warm-blooded, so we have to burn calories to keep our blood warm and to stay alive. The colder your environment is, the more calories your body needs to burn to stay warm. Your body reacts to cold by shivering when exposed to cold. Shivering creates body heat, which helps you burn calories.

Humans have two kinds of adipose (fat) tissue: white and brown. White fat tissue is for energy storage, and brown fat is burned to produce body heat. Regular, long-term exposure to cold will help the body produce more brown fat. Brown adipose tissue burns more calories than white fat and is used to keep the body warm.

Studies show that being in temperatures of 61°F for about two hours a day, resulted in an additional 140 calories burned per day. Being in a lower room temperature daily could increase weight loss by 5-10 pounds per year. As you get used to colder temperatures, you'll begin to shiver less while continuing to burn calories to produce heat. Turning down the thermostat can help with long-term weight loss by increasing your brown fat reserves, as long as you're not compensating by overeating.

23.   Give Yourself a Break

Have some compassion for yourself, because it is a challenge. We live in a toxic food environment of foods scientifically engineered to make you eat more so companies can profit from overconsumption. The food marketing system, including food service and food retailing, supplied about $1.77 trillion worth of food in 2019. Our food environment is built to make it hard for people to eat healthier. You have to swim upstream and against cultural norms to be a healthy eater.

Ernesto Martinez

Expenditures for food at home and away from home

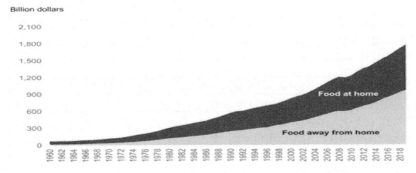

Source: USDA, Economic Research Service using data from the Food Expenditure Series (FES), nominal expenditures.

24. Wear Fitted Clothing

Clothing has two crucial roles in weight loss. First, caring about your appearance is essential for your self-esteem, and dressing well will remind you of your goals. Plus, those beautiful clothes will serve as a visual reminder before a meal to help you keep your goals.

Second, clothes don't directly make you lose weight, but if you wear tight pants all the time, regardless of your initial weight, you'll notice pretty much right away if you start to gain or lose weight. Other examples include wearing a sports bra, so you remember to do exercise that day. Wearing a belt will remind you if you overeat and your belly starts bulging above and below, then you'll be sure to keep your portion sizes in check. Avoid stretchable clothing when you're not exercising. They don't allow you to be aware when your body is expanding, instead wear fitted clothing so you can see and feel the difference when it's easier or harder to get into your jeans.

25. Dress Up to Exercise

Dress for success, even at the gym. Wearing nice clothes boosts your self-esteem, influences positive behavior, and it helps subconsciously change how you act. When you put on fitness clothing, it's like getting into character, and it can make you perform better, making you more mentally prepared for the task. You'll look at yourself in the mirror during your workout, and you'll feel more confident in your abilities, which could improve performance, focus, motivation, and gains. How you look is a reflection of what you eat. Proper clothing for each activity also helps prevent injuries and protect you from the elements. For example, you can wear insulated fabrics for a run in cold weather or breathable, sweat-wicking material to keep your skin cool and dry in hot weather.

In general, if you're not feeling good about yourself, it's hard to get to the gym, because some people feel self-conscious and think others are watching them. Dressing yourself up and even putting on some makeup will make you feel better about yourself.

26. Wear Sport Clothes

Research shows that people who wear sports clothing are more likely to be more physically active. People who go casual at least once a week take an additional 491 steps and burn 25 more calories than when they wore business attire. Going casual just once a week could slash 6,250 calories over the year, enough to prevent the average annual weight gain (0.4 to 1.8 pounds) experienced by most Americans.

27. Keep Your Fridge Stocked

When you get home from work tired and hungry, if you don't have food available, you'll be more likely to order unhealthy take-out food. Cook extra portions of healthy meals and keep them readily available in the fridge in case you are hungry and want something fast. Also, stock healthy frozen and fresh chopped fruits and vegetables so you can whip up a quick vegetable stir fry with frozen veggies and make yourself a delicious fruit smoothie for dessert in minutes. Develop the habit of stocking your fridge and pantry with healthy foods to make losing weight much more straightforward.

28. Size Matters

People who visit the USA often report leaving with a few extra pounds, even Americans who embark on vacation indicate that they come back weighing less. This is due mostly to USA's portion sizes which are 1.5-2 times larger than the rest of the world, not to mention that the US is the world leader in buffets per capita.

Studies show that people consistently eat more food when offered bigger portions. Portion control is essential when you're trying to lose weight and keep it off. Managing your portions doesn't mean you have to go hungry; it means you have to make better food choices.

We need less food and calories as we age. Measure the amounts of food you eat with a measuring cup, spoons, and a measuring scale to help you learn about portion sizes, so you have an idea of how much you need to eat. Commercially available prepackaged portion size meals help you to stay on track eating only the calories that you're supposed to eat to reach your weight goals. Eat pre-portioned foods such as 100 calorie snack packs. Don't eat out of large packages of food because you may munch your way through several servings.

29.   Think Ahead

It's easier to avoid eating foods than it is to burn the fat accumulated by eating the food. Eating a 300 calorie brownie would take walking 3 miles at a 4mph pace to burn the calories off through exercise.

30.   Learn to Cook

Learning how to cook will allow you to save money and avoid restaurant food, which is often high in calories, fat, and sugar. Learning how to prepare meals will help you manage your weight and lose weight without reducing food intake. People who cook are also more likely to eat a wide variety of highly nutritious ingredients, including fruit and vegetables, which promote weight loss. People who do not cook have higher rates of obesity. If you're not sure how to cook, start by watching cooking videos on YouTube.

31.   Choose Healthier Cooking Methods

Frying, broiling, and grilling are amongst the unhealthiest cooking methods available. Although these foods tend to be tasty and calorie-dense, the process creates several types of harmful chemical compounds when cooked under high heat. These compounds include acrylamides, acrolein, advanced glycation end products (AGEs), heterocyclic amines, oxysterols, and polycyclic aromatic hydrocarbons (PAHs). Many of the chemicals formed during high-heat cooking increase your risk of cancer and heart disease. To avoid collateral health damage, choose milder and healthier cooking methods, such as boiling, stewing, steaming, and blanching.

32. Store Away Leftovers

After cooking a meal, serve yourself, store the rest in the fridge, and eat dinner. If you leave your food out on the stove, you're going to want to keep nibbling. Packing away leftovers will keep it fresh for future meals, prevent boredom or mindless eating, and overeating. Try the same strategy when you eat out, bring a storage container (environmentally friendly) or ask for a to-go container along with your meal, that way you can portion out what you want and pack up the rest for later to help prevent overeating.

You can also add extra vegetables and fruit to the leftovers at your next meal to help improve the nutritional content of the food.

33. Avoid Cooking Shows

Cooking shows have become a trend on social media and cable networks. Unfortunately, most of the recipes featured on these media outlets are unhealthy dishes and sweets. Therefore, the internet and social media are helping make people fatter. With the increased time people spend watching social media, the barrage of unhealthy foods makes it impossible to avoid cravings and indulgences. If you notice them, it's best to skip them over.

Studies show that women who watch cooking programs and cook from scratch weigh 11 pounds more than people who watch the programs and don't cook. Although people who cook from scratch are healthier than people who dine out, the difference is cooking shows encourage and teach people to consume indulgent, unhealthy foods.

Women who watch cooking programs, also known as "viewers," weigh an average of 153 pounds, which is higher than the average weight of those who don't view cooking shows. Women who watch and prepare foods made on cooking shows, also known as "doers," weigh even more, on average, 164 pounds. People who watch and try to recreate dishes made on cooking shows take pride in trying to replicate these recipes, making little to no effort in trying to reduce the extra fat and sugar that is typically associated with these programs.

People should be cooking at home, they need to be conscious of the ingredients they're using, and not tempted by the media to eat the worst foods.

34. Learn New Recipes

Family recipes and comfort foods are unique because they taste good and bring back strong, pleasant memories of growing up. On average, the traditional meals your parents and grandparents used to make are much higher in calories and are less compatible with our less-active generation. These meals are best for special occasions, check out healthier recipes for daily use.

35. Avoid Polluted Air

Research has shown that inhaling automobile and diesel exhaust alters signals generated and received by the fat cells. They are causing these cells to grow 12 to 25 percent larger in size and increase in number. The pollution disrupts communication between cells causing inflammation, increased lipid storage, and immune system activation. The inflammation and immune response can trigger further fat cell production, causing a feedback loop where the two systems keep nudging the other forward. Air pollution also disrupts the blood-brain barrier, causing a stroke, Multiple Sclerosis, and neurodegenerative diseases such as Parkinson's Disease and Alzheimer's.

If you live in an area where there are high air pollution levels, or the air quality is low on that day. Limit exposure to air pollution to help you avoid the stress and unbalance it causes to your body. Use an air filter in your home, recirculate the air in the car so your car air filter can clean the air in your cabin, and adjust outdoor activities. Due to the increased respiration rate during exercise, avoid exercising outside during poor air quality days and stay away from roadways, where exposure to these pollutants is higher.

36. Be Mindful of Holiday Weight

Studies show that holiday meals can add an average of one pound of body weight each year and add on additional pounds year after year. So even though most of us think we'll work the weight off after the holidays, it doesn't usually work out that way. Around the holidays, keep in mind that it's much harder to lose weight than it is to prevent gaining it. Aside from all of the strategies in this book, try making low-fat versions of traditional dishes around the holidays to avoid creeping weight gain over time.

37. Prime Yourself for Weight Loss

When you're hungry, your willpower will be at its weakest, your cravings the strongest, and you're most likely to make the worst food selections. Your subconscious mind is full of memories of unhealthy foods that gave you pleasant experiences in the past, like pizza, danish, or whatever else you find appealing. These foods are stimulating because of their high sugar, salt, and fat content. So your brain saves memories of the images and feelings you had when you ate them.

When you're hungry, these images of high-calorie foods will start flashing through your mind, your mouth will start watering, you'll start feeling some of the same pleasure you felt when you ate them, and you'll crave eating those foods. For this reason, people who rely on willpower to lose weight will eventually give up and put the weight back on.

Priming is a technique to help people get rid of cravings for the unhealthiest foods they crave most. If, for example, your goal is to decrease your sugar intake, then use negative priming. Watch documentaries or read books about how lousy overeating sugar is for your weight. When you attempt to eat sugar, you'll recall those terrible images and negative information, and your desire to eat the food will decrease. You can use this same technique for processed foods, fast foods, meats, desserts, smoking, alcohol, or any other habit you're trying to break. Priming helps you eat healthier, learn positive habits, or break bad ones.

An example of positive priming would be if you don't like eating vegetables and your goal was to increase your veggie intake. Then watch YouTube videos on the benefits of eating more veggies. Your brain will start filling its' memory banks with this information and when you're at the grocery deciding which foods to buy. Your mind will flash images of delicious-looking vegetable dishes, skinny people, and a lower body weight number on the scale. The reprogramming will replace the old memories of junk food that gave you pleasure and caused weight gain with new mental images that will help you make the desired choice.

38.   Variety is the Spice of Life

Including various fruits and vegetables in your diet is one of the best ways to obtain the antioxidants, vitamins, and minerals you need. Even if you don't like all types of fruits and vegetables, the more diversity, the better, that's because each food offers a unique blend of nutrients, especially beneficial antioxidants and phytonutrients. Even different foods from within the same food group provide a diverse mix of nutrients. Switching things up is an excellent way to ensure you're covering all your bases.

It's already difficult enough for most people to stick to a healthy diet long term, but when repeating the same meals over and over again starts to feel uninspiring and restrictive, this can make things even more challenging. You might start feeling like you're eating on autopilot, which means mindless eating and cravings are more likely to occur.

If you don't enjoy the things you're eating and you start feeling deprived, you're very unlikely to gain any benefits from your diet long term. Eventually, you'll fall off the wagon and decide you require more fun and flavor. To make healthy eating something you can sustain, focus on trying new things, such as different seasonal fruits, vegetables, and grains.

When you expose yourself to lots of different food groups, you're more likely to develop a greater diversity of healthy bacteria in your gut. Bacterial diversity is associated with benefits, including protection against obesity, reduced allergies, and enhanced immunity.

Eating various fats and proteins is also essential for obtaining a mix of fatty acids and amino acids, vital for functions like cholesterol balance, cognitive health, mood stabilization, connective tissue healing, and much more.

39.　Honesty is the Best Policy

Be Honest with yourself. No dietitian, physician, therapist, or nurse can be with you 24 hours a day to advise or monitor you on what you should be eating. The best strategy is to be accountable to yourself, monitor your behavior, and coach yourself when you realize you can do better. To lose weight, you have to be completely honest with yourself.

Ask yourself, are you really keeping track of everything you eat? Are you slipping a few extra treats and snacks? Some of the most common excuses patients make when they don't meet their weight loss goals include, "I really don't eat that much." "I eat really healthy." "I'm gaining weight because my knees are bad, and I can't exercise." "I think I have a hormone problem." "I'm gaining weight because I couldn't get an appointment to see the nutritionist." "I have big bones." "I am doing everything I was told to do, but the recommendations are just not working for me!" Be honest with yourself. It's easy to find excuses for not losing weight. If you want to know how to honestly lose weight, don't allow yourself to exaggerate your challenges and turn minor obstacles into excuses for failure. It comes down to respect. Do you respect yourself enough to be completely honest with yourself?

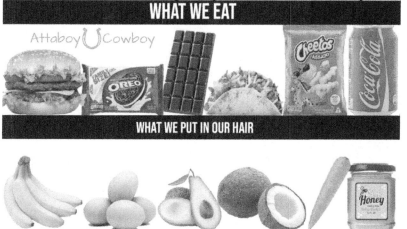

40. Keep It Simple

The harder and more time consuming you make something, the less likely you are to keep up with it. Switching to a new routine takes an initial time investment, which causes some people to give up, and order high-calorie takeout. You don't have to cut gourmet food or keep up with the latest trends to lose weight. Keep it simple. Instead, find a few favorite healthy, go-to recipes and stick to them.

41. Meditation

Meditation takes many forms, including mindfulness meditation, repeating a mantra, guided imagery, or visualization. By reducing the sympathetic nervous system's anxiety-inducing fight or flight response, meditation can decrease your heart rate, lower your blood pressure, relax your muscles, and slow your breathing. Meditation also structurally changes the brain's cerebral cortex, which plays an instrumental role in memory, attention, and consciousness. Meditation can treat anxiety, stress, chronic pain, depression, and cancer. The psychological benefits include increased emotional stability, calmness, decreased anxiety, and greater self-confidence.

Meditation, especially mindfulness meditation, can be an essential component of your weight loss plan. Over time, it can help you make lasting changes to your thought patterns, eating habits, and even how you feel about your weight.

B. Weight Loss Treatments

42. Acupuncture

An acupuncturist inserts hair-thin needles at specific body points or energy pathways to restore the flow of qi. The needles stimulate acupoints, which cause the nervous system to release opium-like endorphins to the muscles, spinal cord, and brain. These chemicals reduce the pain experience and trigger the release of other chemicals and hormones that influence the body's internal regulating system. Creating a calming effect counteracting excessive eating caused by increased stress, anxiety, or frustration. In this respect, acupuncture can calm those afflicted and help them lose weight without resorting to drugs. Acupuncture represents an efficient complementary and alternative medical therapeutic option for obesity control.

43. Acupressure

Acupressure practitioners (can be applied to oneself) use tools or their hands to apply pressure to specific acupoints on the body to open energy flows, promote emotional balance, and release tension. Stimulating various points in the body can trigger the release of endorphins, the body's pain-reducing chemicals that increase blood flow and oxygen to areas of the body to relieve discomfort and soreness. Acupressure reduces stress, boosts digestion, and improves metabolism, all of which play a role in weight management.

44. Aromatherapy

Aromatic essential oils are extracted from plants, distilled, and mixed with other substances such as alcohol or lotion. They are then applied to the skin for absorption or sprayed into the air for inhaling. Inhaling a scent triggers powerful neurotransmitters and other chemicals that stimulate certain parts of the limbic system, which control emotions and behavior, resulting in an improved mood. Aromatherapy, also known as essential oil therapy, can enhance both physical and emotional health. Some of the benefits offered by aromatherapy include:

- reduce anxiety
- relieve tension
- reduce feelings of depression
- ease aches and pains in the body
- improve digestion
- curb food cravings
- energize your workout
- correct cellulite
- correct stretch marks

45. Flower Essence

In the 1930s, Dr. Edward Bach created the flower essence system. Flower therapy, or essence therapy, is considered vibrational medicine, based on the idea that everything in nature, including flowers and your own body, has its own vibration. When vibration is out of tune in the body, which can be caused by emotional distress and illness, using flower essences with its specific vibration can help restore calm and balance.

Distilled essences of wildflowers, which are liquids infused with a flower's energy, are usually preserved in an alcohol base and administered internally, under the tongue, to balance your emotions. The goal in vibrational medicine is to move, unblock or balance life energy over the physical, energetic, and spiritual body. Doing so will help bring about mental, physical, and spiritual wellness.

Flower essences are water-based, made only from flowers. On the other hand, aromatherapy essential oils are oil-based and made from the aromatic parts of plants. The main difference is flower essences are typically taken internally with an eyedropper. You can add them to your water bottle and sip throughout the day. In contrast, essential oils are applied topically or inhaled.

46. Hydrotherapy

Hydrotherapy is also known as aquatic therapy, water

therapy, pool therapy, and balneotherapy. Water is used externally or internally in different forms (water, ice, steam) to promote or treat various diseases with various temperatures, pressure, duration, and site. Hydrotherapy improves many health disorders, including; immunity, manages pain, cardiac problems, respiratory issues, circulatory disorders, fatigue, anxiety, obesity, hypercholesterolemia, labor, and hyperthermia. The results vary depending on the temperature of the water and how it is applied.

47. Massage

Massage effectively reduces symptoms such as stress, pain, anxiety, depression, nausea, and fatigue in people who have had chemotherapy or surgery for cancer. Deep tissue massage encourages lymphatic flow and circulation, which aid in detoxification and weight loss. Along with a natural whole foods diet, massage can help reduce excess fat and weight in your body.

48. Hyperbaric Chamber

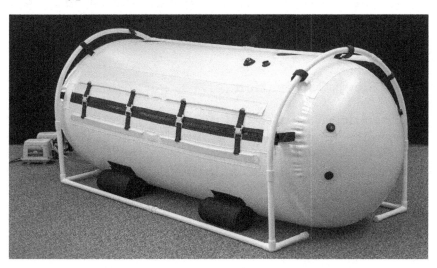

Hyperbaric oxygen therapy (HBOT) accelerates the healing process of almost any medical disorder.

You enter a chamber with pressure levels of 1.5 to 3

times higher than average, relax, sit, or lie comfortably and breathe in pure oxygen using a mask. Oxygen is forced into the blood, infusing the injured tissues that need more oxygen so that they can begin healing and restore healthy body function.

HBOT prevents "reperfusion injury," which is tissue damage that happens when blood supply returns to tissues after being deprived of oxygen. Damaged cells start releasing harmful free radicals into the body. Free radicals damage body tissues, cause the blood vessels to clamp up, and stop blood flow. HBOT helps the body's oxygen radical scavengers to find the problem molecules and assist healing to continue.

HBOT helps block harmful bacteria from releasing toxins into the body and strengthens the body's immune system. It also increases the concentration of oxygen in the tissues, which fight infections, and helps white blood cells find and destroy invaders.

HBOT promotes the formation of new collagen, blood vessels, and skin cells. It also stimulates cells to produce vascular endothelial growth factor, which attracts and stimulates endothelial cells necessary for healing.

For faster results HBOT can be used at least three times a week or twice a day for optimal outcomes.

C. Sleep Issues

49. Sleep Deprivation

Sleep deprivation can cause weight gain, decreased life expectancy, and disrupt essential hormones involved in metabolism. People who work the night shift are more susceptible to weight gain because you're less likely to refuse foods when you're tired and are more vulnerable to over-eating After sleeping only 4 hours a day for six days straight, people were unable to regulate their blood sugar properly, leading to overeating due to feelings of hunger. Lack of sleep makes you susceptible to heart disease, diabetes, stroke, cancer, high blood pressure, and a weaker immune system. Your mortality rate will also increase exponentially. Getting 7-8 hours a day will help you keep your blood sugar in check, maintain weight, and prevent binge eating.

Middle-aged women naturally see a decrease in their estrogen levels, which affects their sleep-wake cycle. This process has the dual effect of decreasing sleep and making it harder to sleep. Sleep deprivation will lower the production of leptin levels, which means you don't register the feeling of fullness that signals you to stop eating. It also raises ghrelin levels, which will make you very hungry. Having this imbalance will make you hungrier for high-calorie, high carb foods. Lack of sleep would affect the function of both hormones.

Lack of sleep can also reduce insulin sensitivity, which means your body is making it, but it's not registering it. Insulin helps your body cells use sugar (glucose) for fuel and also converts calories into fat. As your body becomes less sensitive, your pancreas has to release higher insulin levels into your bloodstream to make sure your cells get enough glucose and keep your blood sugar regular. The extra insulin causes calories to get stored as fat. If you're older, that excess fat gets stored in your abdomen. Studies have shown a correlation between lack of sleep and increased BMI. Eighty percent of adults who are chronically sleep-deprived, average four or more health problems.

50. Factors to Help Improve Sleep

- Stick to a sleeping schedule, go to sleep and wake up at the same time every day. The duration, timing, and quality of your sleep will help keep your hormones balanced.
- Try an iPhone sleep application designed to help you maximize your sleep, such as sleep cycle, sleep coach, or sonic.
- Excessive ambient light can adversely affect your sleep-wake cycle. Decrease the lighting in your bedroom as you get closer to bedtime and install light-blocking shades for the mornings if necessary to prolong your sleep. Unplug or place a piece of

black electrical tape on electronics that emit light in your bedroom, such as televisions, blue or red lights on electronic devices, and lay your cell phone facedown.

- Switch your bedroom light bulbs from CFLs and LEDs to halogen. Reducing the amount of exposure to blue light will improve your sleep. Excess blue light causes inflammation and mitochondrial dysfunction and affects glucose control, leading to high blood sugar and increases in insulin resistance.

- Using red light in the evenings will help your body transition into its sleep cycle more naturally. Right before going to bed, switch to red lights in your bedroom, the low color temperature will have a soothing effect on your body, and it's the most conducive wavelength of light for a good night's sleep.

- As you age, we need more bathroom breaks during the night. So install night lights so you can go to the bathroom without turning on the overhead lights, which can make it harder to go back to sleep. In the mornings, open the shades to let the light in, which helps regulate your sleep patterns.

- If you're having problems sleeping, set up a camera in your room to record your sleeping and help you figure out if you have sleep apnea. Sleep apnea can be a severe sleep disorder in which breathing repeatedly stops and starts throughout the night. If you feel tired after a full night's sleep and snore, you may have sleep apnea. Obstructed breathing can cause you to wake you up hundreds of times throughout the night, and push your hormones levels out of balance.

- Excessive exercise with inadequate rest increases susceptibility to infections, decreases the body's ability to heal, alter sleep patterns and hormonal patterns, and increases circulating levels of the stress hormone cortisol.

51. Avoid Day Time Naps

Research has determined that people burn fewer calories when they sleep during the day and stay up at night. Sleeping during the day will cause you to burn 52 to 59 fewer calories because your circadian rhythm is off, affecting the metabolism to malfunction. If your circadian rhythm is off, spending a weekend in the wilderness can help it get back on track.

52. Ditch the Alarm Clock

Being shocked out of bed by a jarring sound can activate your sympathetic nervous system. Increasing your blood pressure and heart rate and adding to your stress levels by getting your adrenaline rushing. The solution to this unhealthy problem is to try gradually waking up to natural light. On average natural risers feel 10 percent more well-rested during the day than people who use an alarm to wake up. They also take less time to feel fully awake than people who need an alarm.

If you aren't able to naturally wake up, try using sounds that won't impact your mood. Use calming sounds rather than an aggressive tune. The ideal alarm or wake-up cues elicit a gentle, relatively gradual shift from deeper to lighter sleep, allowing a more natural, less stressful awakening.

Try to wake up gradually using progressively intensifying sounds that advance from very soft to louder. Even graded exposure to light tends to work best to induce the gradual changes in brain activity that mimic natural awakening. Some of the best sounds to use are; raindrops, sounds of a rainforest, your favorite song, water (ocean waves, streams, or rivers), smooth jazz, birds singing, soft musical instruments (flutes, harps, violins, and pianos), and the sound of crickets.

53. Adjust your Sleep

Researchers at the University of Southern California (USC) found that people who slept 6 1/2 hours a night on average lived longer than people who slept eight hours a day. The amount of sleep your body needs depends on the lifestyle you live. For example, higher amounts of stress, poor eating habits, or lack of exercise will cause you to sleep more. Eating healthier, exercising, not smoking, or drinking will cause your body to take on less damage and require less recovery time through sleep.

If you went out the night before for drinks, ate unhealthy food, or didn't sleep well last night. Adjust your behavior the following day. Eat healthier, exercise less than usual, and avoid stressful situations. When your body is not well-rested, these three factors can do more damage to your body than expected.

54. Treat Snoring

Almost half of all American adults snore. Snoring happens when air cannot move air freely through your nose and throat during sleep. Having excess floppy throat and nasal tissue will cause the tissue to vibrate and produce the familiar snoring sound. Snoring can disrupt your sleep or that of your partner and be a sign of a health condition, including:

Obesity

Obstructive sleep apnea (blocked airways)

Sleep deprivation

Structural abnormality of your nose, mouth, or throat

Consumption of alcohol too close to bedtime

Improper positioning such as sleeping on your back

Snoring interrupts your sleep, leading to fatigue, which makes you hungrier and less active leading to weight gain. Over the long term, snoring alters your metabolism, increases your appetite, and decreases energy expenditure. Snoring can cause obesity, and obesity can cause snoring.

Over 70% of patients with sleep apnea are obese, and 40% of obese people have sleep apnea. Excess fat around the neck causes compression of the upper airway, especially when lying down, increasing snoring. Midriff fat around the chest compresses the ribcage, which worsens snoring and sleep apnea. Belly fat pushes your diaphragm up, shrinking the volume of your lungs and restricting airflow and air needed to keep some shape in the throat to prevent collapse. Therefore, weight loss is the most effective way to get rid of snoring and sleep apnea.

Men are more likely to snore because they tend to gain weight around their neck, chest, and abdomen. While women usually gain body fat peripherally: on the thighs, butt, and hips.

Snoring can decrease your blood oxygen levels, which strains your brain and organs while doubling your risk of developing diabetes, obesity, and high blood pressure. If you have sleep apnea, your risk goes up 70 to 80%. People can half the effects of sleep apnea by losing only 10-15% of their body weight.

Chronic sleep deprivation caused by snoring or sleep apnea makes you tired, less energy to exercise, and triggers cravings for high sugar foods to boost your energy. So, while you may think you're hungry, you may be sleep-deprived. More snoring produces worse sleep and more exhaustion, which in turn is mitigated by overeating and under-exercising.

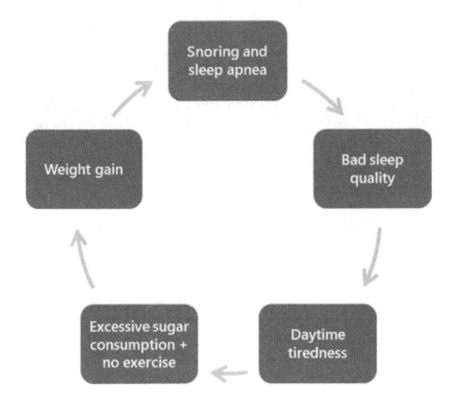

55.   Have a Sleep Study

Polysomnography, commonly known as a sleep study, is a test used to diagnose sleep disorders. During a Polysomnography, you go into a sleep disorder unit within a hospital or sleep center. Once dressed in comfortable clothing, you lay down to sleep in a comfortable bed with a camera recording your entire sleep study. Sensors are also placed on your body to record your brain waves, heart rate, breathing, and oxygen levels in your blood, as well as eye and leg movements during the study. The test records your sleep stages and cycles to identify if your sleep patterns are disrupted and why.

Common reasons for a sleep study:

- Periodic limb movement disorder sometimes associated with restless leg syndrome. In this sleep disorder, you involuntarily extend and flex your legs while sleeping.

- Sleep apnea or other sleep-related breathing disorders. In this condition, your breathing repeatedly starts and stops during sleep.

- Narcolepsy is a chronic sleep disorder that causes overwhelming daytime drowsiness and sudden attacks of sleep.

- Unexplained chronic insomnia is characterized by consistent trouble falling asleep or staying asleep.

- Unusual behaviors during sleep are characterized by unusual activities during sleep, such as moving around a lot, walking, or rhythmic movements.

- Rapid eye movement (REM) sleep behavior disorder is characterized by acting out dreams as you sleep.

D. Digestive Issues

56. Reduce stress

When you get stressed, the executive control system in the brain, which is the signal to stop eating, becomes exhausted. Therefore stopping yourself from doing things you want becomes more difficult and energy-intense. So when you're stressed, there isn't as much energy dedicated to stopping your impulses to eat.

Increased stress levels can also cause hormonal imbalance. When under stress, your body produces hormones called glucocorticoids. Increased levels of glucocorticoids can increase a person's appetite, causing weight gain. Cortisol is a type of glucocorticoid; higher levels of stress will create higher levels of cortisol in your body, causing you to take in more calories. Stress can also precipitate emotional eating, which involves eating unhealthful foods to control and improve a negative mood. Strategies for reducing stress include regular exercise, sex, reducing caffeine intake, practicing meditation or mindfulness, spending time outdoors, and saying no to non-essential commitments.

Controlling stress helps decrease weight by preventing stress eating and the release of hormones that cause weight gain. It's your perception and handling of an event and not the nature of the stressor, that determines its effect on you. The more control you perceive yourself to have over a stressful situation, the less damaging the stress will be.

People under stress snack more and tend to crave sugary and fatty foods like chips and cookies, which can add to belly fat quickly. Stressed people want sweet foods because they cause you to release endorphins, which act as a drug to calm stress, make you feel good, and improve mood. But eating sweets can cause a sugar crash afterward, causing more cravings and causing you to eat more.

Take control of stress by identifying long term stressors

and relieving tension with non-caloric treats.

Develop a list of non-food activities to combat stress and to use when you're stressed. For example, getting a massage, buying flowers, gardening, playing video games, watching a movie, talking to a friend, or family member are non-food activities to participate in. Exercise is the best option as it lowers stress and helps you drop weight.

57.   Protein

Protein is necessary for growth, an efficient metabolism, increasing feelings of fullness, and delaying hunger. It also plays a role in reversing age-related muscle loss which helps you build muscle and burn calories, and because it also takes more calories to break down and digest proteins, it also reduces weight.

Eating protein for snacks reduces calorie intake at later meals. Eating eggs for breakfast will cause you to eat fewer calories at lunch compared to those who ate a grain-based breakfast. You'll also eat fewer calories for the next 36 hours.

A simple way to increase protein intake is to add a tablespoon of chia seeds or hemp seeds to your meals.

Eat protein with every meal. If you're craving sweets after a meal, then you are not eating enough protein. Not eating enough protein can lead to weight gain and cause you to eat foods such as sugars that will cause weight gain.

Some examples of protein-rich foods include lean meats, greek yogurt, legumes, quinoa, and nuts.

58.   Spread your Protein Consumption Out

Most Americans eat very little protein for breakfast, moderate amounts for lunch, and high amounts of protein for dinner. For optimal protein synthesis, distribute your protein intake evenly throughout the day. Researchers have found that people who spread their protein throughout the day, absorb 25% more protein overall.

59. Be Aware of Food Allergies

Burping or passing gas after a meal means you're either eating too fast or eating too many foods that your body has a problem digesting. You could have food intolerance or allergies. Foods such as soy, gluten, dairy, or refined grains can cause inflammation, a weakened immune system, bloating, and weight gain. Over time, eating foods that you have a hard time digesting will lead to these foods building up in your gut along with gas and fluids. This process slows down your metabolism and leads to more weight gain. If you're not sure which foods are upsetting your stomach, use a food journal to keep track of the foods you eat or try an elimination diet.

60. Indigestion

Overeating can cause indigestion. As your stomach fills with foods that it cannot digest, your body tries to deal with this by producing more acid to break it down. As the acid builds up it starts to overflow into your esophagus resulting in acid reflux. This process causes inflammation, bloating, weight gain, and a slower metabolism.

61. Regular Bowel Movements

Regular bowel movements that resemble a brown banana means your immune system is working properly. Variations such as slimy, pebble-like consistency, yellow, watery, mucusy, or requiring strong pushing, grunting, excessive amounts of time, or sweating all mean you're not eating a balanced diet. Incomplete or not consistently defecating will allow waste to build up inside your body. Accumulating waste in your intestinal tract can lead to aging, poor intestinal health, and weight gain. Going multiple times a day to the restroom is a sign of good health, but the minimum should be once a day. Food that is not evacuated can sit over a week at a time in your gut, decaying and releasing toxins into your body instead of simply releasing nutrients when it's fresh inside your body.

This process can slow your metabolism, lead to weight gain secondary to waste sitting in your intestines, bloating, and cause multiple health problems.

62.   Laxatives

Laxatives should be used in emergency situations. If you're using them more than twice a year, then you are not eating properly. Laxatives rush food through your intestinal tract, preventing your body from absorbing the nutrients it needs from the food you eat. Taking laxatives will slow your metabolism, cause weight gain, cause vitamin and mineral deficiencies, cause problems losing weight, and lead to premature aging. If you're not able to defecate naturally, you have to address problems related to not eating properly, a medical issue, or an eating disorder.

63.   Hair Loss

Hair loss is a sign of poor circulation and slow metabolism, which will lead to weight gain. Multiple issues can cause hair loss, but not all of them cause weight gain, therefore, it is vital to explore whether your weight gain is related to not eating properly, genetics, a medical issue, or an eating disorder.

E. Condiments

64. Try Healthy Condiments

Condiments are an excellent option for adding flavor to food, cutting calories, and enhancing health benefits. However, be mindful of unhealthy ingredients such as vegetable oils, trans fats, artificial additives, and excessive amounts of sugar or salt. Some condiments are so unhealthy that they can turn a healthy meal into an unhealthy one.

Healthy Options

- **Salsa**

Salsa is now more popular as a condiment than ketchup in the US. Salsa is packed with health benefits from onion, garlic, tomatoes, cilantro, and chili peppers. Additionally, it's very low in calories; two tablespoons of salsa has only ten calories, versus ranch dressing which has 119 calories. Fresh salsa is ideal since the vegetables will retain most of their healthy properties. If you buy ready-made salsa, check the ingredients and avoid salsas with high amounts of added sugar.

- **Hot Sauce**

One of the healthiest condiments available is hot sauce. It's very versatile, adds a lot of flavors, and only has six calories per teaspoon. Additionally, capsaicin, a compound found in chili peppers, accelerates your metabolism, is an anti-inflammatory, and increases weight loss.

- **Guacamole**

Guacamole is a superfood salad made by combining mashed avocado, onion, jalapeño, garlic, cilantro, lime juice, and salt. The high fiber and healthy fat content will help keep you satiated for long periods.

- **Pesto**

Pesto is made of fresh basil leaves, parmesan cheese, extra virgin olive oil, and pine nuts. Because it is raw, pesto sauce is high in zinc and several other nutrients.

- **Mustard**

There are many varieties of mustard made from mustard seeds, distilled vinegar, garlic powder, turmeric, lemon juice, and salt. Mustard has only six calories per two teaspoons. The ingredients in mustard are anti-inflammatory and provide a variety of health benefits.

- **Raw Honey**

Raw honey is unpasteurized and minimally processed making it richer in nutrients in comparison to commercially made honey. Raw honey has antioxidants that prevent cellular damage, as well as anti-inflammatory and antibacterial compounds.

- **Tahini**

Tahini is a middle eastern sauce made from ground sesame seeds. Sesame seeds are rich in zinc, selenium, copper, iron, and vitamin B6 that support thyroid health and helps to stabilize weight. It also has five grams of protein for every two teaspoons.

- **Grass-Fed Butter**

Compared to regular butter, grass-fed butter contains over 500% more of the fatty acid conjugated linoleic acid (CLA), which promotes weight loss. Grass-fed butter is rich in good cholesterol, omega-3 fats, saturated fats, vitamins A, D, E, K2, and iodine, lecithin, and selenium. It is also anti-inflammatory and helps fight heart disease. However, because more land is needed for grass-fed animals to graze, the products are less sustainable and cause more damage to the environment.

- **Plain Greek Yogurt**

Plain Greek yogurt doesn't contain added sugar and is a healthy alternative to most cream-based condiments. Greek yogurt is a low-calorie substitute for mayonnaise or sour cream and is high in calcium and protein. Seven ounces of low-fat Greek yogurt contains nearly 20 grams of protein, reduces hunger, and promotes muscle growth.

- **Apple Cider Vinegar**

Apple cider vinegar helps improve blood sugar control after a meal, which is helpful for diabetes, and a good alternative for salad dressing.

- **Nutritional Yeast**

Nutritional yeast is a nutritious vegan alternative for cheese. It's high in protein, vitamins, minerals, and antioxidants. Nutritional yeast protects against oxidative damage, lowers cholesterol, and boosts immunity.

- **Sauerkraut**

Sauerkraut is made from fermented cabbage and is high in dietary fiber and contains vitamins C and K, potassium, calcium, and phosphorus. Sauerkraut has over 28 different probiotic strains and is very beneficial for gut health.

- **Kimchi**

Kimchi is a Korean condiment made from fermented cabbage, garlic, onion, chili pepper, and salt. It is a rich source of good bacteria. These healthy bacteria live in your gut and improve cholesterol levels, your immune system, skin health, and increase weight loss.

- **Nut Butter**

Nut butter such as almond, cashew, hazelnut, and peanut butter are high in minerals, healthy fats, and protein, two tablespoons have an average of 7 grams. They increase satiety and aid blood sugar regulation and weight management.

- **Tamari**

Tamari is a Japanese sauce similar to soy sauce and made from fermented soybeans. Tamari has a darker appearance, thicker texture, richer flavor, and 45% more protein than traditional soy sauce. Two tablespoons of tamari provide almost 4 grams of protein and is gluten-free.

- **Lemon Juice**

Lemon juice is an adaptable and healthy condiment that is rich in vitamin C, a powerful antioxidant, and is low in sugar. It benefits your skin, immune system, heart health, burns fat, and boosts weight loss.

- **Balsamic Vinegar**

Balsamic vinegar is made from aged grapes. It's rich in antioxidants, especially polyphenol antioxidants like flavonoids, caffeic acid, and gallic acid. These antioxidants protect against cell damage and prevent oxidation of LDL (bad) cholesterol, which can lower your risk of heart disease.

- **Extra Virgin Olive Oil**

Extra virgin olive oil is made from the first pressing of olives and is minimally processed. Olive oil supports heart health and reduces inflammation. Due to its rich antioxidant content, it helps reduce cell damage in your body. Extra virgin olive oil should be consumed raw to preserve its nutritional compounds. We need a steady intake of polyunsaturated oils in our diet because they are the building blocks of eicosanoids. Eicosanoids are a powerful hormone that controls every cell, organ, and system in our body. These hormones will dictate how well your immune system works, whether you lose weight, have pain and inflammation, or have a heart attack.

- **Toasted Sesame Oil**

Toasted sesame oil is produced by toasting sesame

seeds before extracting the oil from them. It has a richer flavor than regular sesame oil and should be used drizzled over foods, instead of for cooking. Sesame oil is an anti-inflammatory, reduces LDL (bad) cholesterol levels, and benefits your heart, joints, skin, and hair.

- **Hummus**

Hummus is a blend of tahini, chickpeas, olive oil, garlic, lemon juice, and salt. Hummus is high in protein, fiber, magnesium, and folate. It's a cocktail of healthy ingredients that help you feel satiated and promotes weight loss.

Unhealthy Condiments to Limit

Many condiments contain artificial chemicals, colors, and sweeteners, and unhealthy oils. They also can contain more calories than the meal itself, so it's essential to be mindful of what you're using and what's inside of it.

- **Ketchup**

Ketchup has four grams of sugar and 190 milligrams of sodium per tablespoon. Eating eight tablespoons of ketchup will have you reaching your sodium needs for the entire day. Because it's also very acidic, it can damage the enamel of your teeth. Luckily, there are healthier versions available that are low sodium, organic, made with fruit juice instead of high fructose corn syrup.

- **Ranch or Thousand Island Dressing**

Ranch dressing is one of the unhealthiest condiments available with a combination of artificial ingredients and is high in calories with two tablespoons providing 129 calories. Thousand island dressing has 111 calories but is higher in sugar with 4.6 grams per two tablespoons. Try small serving sizes or better yet use a lower-calorie alternative like salsa or a salad dressing made from wholesome, low-sugar ingredients.

- **Margarine**

Margarine is tricky because most of their packaging has several health claims, and they prey on the publics' belief that butter is not good for you. The product is typically made with unhealthy vegetable oils, trans fats, and has traces of healthy oil like olive oil, which allows advertisers to claim the benefits of that healthy oil. Most margarines cause inflammation and heart damage. Use healthy fats like grass-fed butter, avocado oil, or extra virgin olive oil instead.

- **Pancake Syrup**

Pancake syrup is a Frankenfood with high sodium, high-fructose corn syrup (HFCS), and usually made exclusively of chemicals produced in laboratories. It causes obesity, heart disease, and type 2 diabetes. Try real fruit, honey, or maple syrup as an alternative.

- **Barbecue Sauce**

BBQ sauce has a lot of added sugar, with two tablespoons containing about 12 to 17 grams. It also has 45 to 70 calories for a two-tablespoon serving and 200 to 350 milligrams of sodium; that's about 14 percent of your daily needs.

- **Teriyaki Sauce**

Teriyaki sauce contains soy sauce, honey or sugar, and sake or mirin (rice wine with less alcohol and more sugar). However, the teriyaki sauce Americans eat is high in sodium, with just two tablespoons providing over 60% of a day's allowance, and high fructose corn syrup. Teriyaki sauce causes inflammation and weight gain. Try making your own teriyaki sauce so that you can use only high-quality ingredients.

- **Monosodium Glutamate (MSG)**

Monosodium glutamate (MSG) is a flavor enhancer used in Chinese food, seasonings, canned vegetables, soups, and processed foods. MSG comes from glutamic acid, an amino acid found in your body, and most foods. It is a popular food additive because it's inexpensive, and it's a powerful flavor enhancer. It has been used for many years because it's considered safe. However, some people's bodies react to it, and some of the symptoms include:

- o Inflammation
- o Headache
- o Weight gain
- o Flushing
- o Sweating
- o Runny nose or congestion
- o Rapid, fluttering heartbeats (heart palpitations)
- o Depression and mood swings
- o Chest pain
- o Upset stomach
- o Fatigue
- o Facial pressure or tightness
- o Body numbness, tingling, or burning
- o Weakness
- o Nausea
- o Hives

Because MSG can be problematic for some people, the FDA requires that products that contain it be labeled. However, because of its low cost and addictive flavor, food companies will often get around some of the labeling requirements by listing the ingredients separately.

Hidden Names for MSG And Free Glutamic Acid:

Ingredients that contain processed free glutamic acid:

- o Glutamate (E 620)
- o Glutamic Acid (E 620)2
- o Monosodium Glutamate (E 621)
- o Monopotassium Glutamate (E 622)
- o Calcium Glutamate (E 623)
- o Monoammonium Glutamate (E 624)
- o Magnesium Glutamate (E 625)
- o Natrium Glutamate

- **Cheese Sauce**

Most cheese sauces such as nacho cheese sauce contain a collection of laboratory-made ingredients like monosodium glutamate (MSG), partially hydrogenated oil, artificial colors, and very little, if any, dairy cheese. The ingredients in cheese sauce are associated with weight gain and inflammation. Try using real unadulterated cheese or nutritional yeast as a replacement.

- **Pasta Sauce**

Store-bought pasta sauces are packed full of artificial ingredients, sugar salt, and fat. Plus, store-bought sauces don't have much fiber, and they're never as nutritious as something you'd make at home.

Canned tomatoes are especially harmful because their acidity is so high that it draws out the bisphenol A (BPA) straight into the contents. Also, a serving of pasta sauce contains more than 35g of sugar.

The convenience is costing you your health. Read the ingredients on the pasta sauce bottles and buy better quality sauces. Marinara sauce typically has minimal ingredients so that you can add your own to it. Or make your own sauce. It's quick, affordable, easy to do, and can make for a very healthy meal.

- **Mayonnaise**

Mayonnaise is a polarizing condiment and one of the most popular for Americans. It's a high-fat food, with no fiber, and made mostly of oil and eggs.

Mayonnaise contains oil, egg yolk, lemon juice or vinegar, and often some mustard. Eighty percent of mayonnaise is oil. The problem is most mayo contains low-quality oils such as soybean or canola oil, which are highly inflammatory. One tablespoon also contains 100 calories, so it's very calorie-dense.

However, mayonnaise can be a healthy option if eaten in moderation and if you choose better quality mayo, such as mayo made with coconut or avocado oil. Avoid mayonnaise made with all other types of fats, as well as low-calorie mayonnaise, which is high in sugar and other artificial ingredients to make up for the loss of taste due to decreased flavor from oil.

65.   Ask for All Condiments on the Side

A condiment is a preparation, sauce, or spice that is added to food to give a specific flavor, enhance the character, or complement the dish.

Condiments sometimes have more calories than the dish itself and are often packed with fat, empty calories, sugar, and artificial ingredients. By asking for the sauce or dressing on the side, you have more control over how much of it you eat, and you could easily save yourself a few hundred calories. By routinely making this request, you could develop a healthy habit to cut calories out of meals.

66.   Pick Red over White Sauce

White sauces are loaded with cream, butter, cheese, and inflammatory oils. While red sauces are made of tomato, vegetables, and often have fewer calories and sugar compared to white sauces. Red sauce is also much higher in healthy vitamins and minerals. On the other hand, the white sauce has a lot of calcium and protein but is high in cholesterol and saturated fat. The red sauce is a healthier alternative than white sauce.

67.   Learn About Sugar so that You Can Avoid it

Sugar, like fat, gives food flavor, which is why it is one of the most commonly added additives to processed food. Because food producers know that people are actively trying to avoid sugar, they use several different types of sugar so they can hide the amount added to foods. Sugar may not be one of the first three ingredients listed, yet the food can still be high in sugar. One of the most common tricks is adding several types of sugars to the same product. Allowing them to have all of the sugars listed further down the ingredient list, but still have high amounts of sugar in the food. So if you were to read the ingredient list, you might think the item is low in sugar, because you don't see the sugars listed high on the list. Food manufacturers like sugar because it is addictive, and if they can get you addicted to their products, then you're going to buy more and help produce more profits for the company.

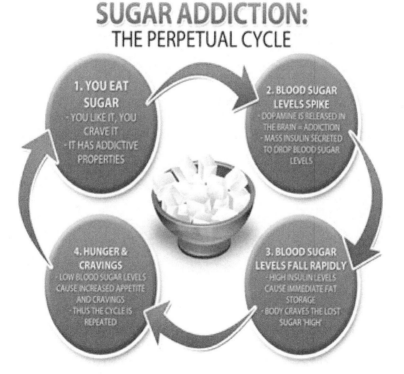

SUGAR ADDICTION:
THE PERPETUAL CYCLE

Most commonly used sweeteners

Types of sugar: evaporated cane juice, beet sugar, cane sugar, brown sugar, buttered sugar, golden sugar, caster sugar, raspadura sugar, coconut sugar, date sugar, invert sugar, muscovado sugar, confectioner's sugar, and organic raw sugar.

Types of syrup: high-fructose corn syrup (one of the worst sugars on the market), rice syrup, carob syrup, maple syrup, golden syrup, agave nectar, malt syrup, honey, oat syrup, and rice bran syrup.

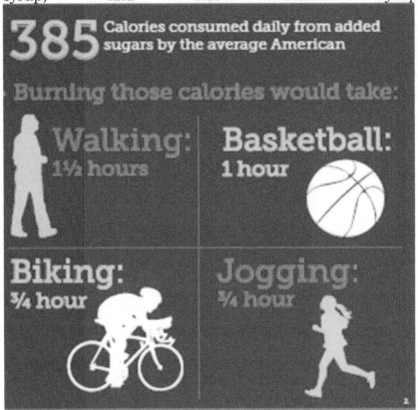

Other sugars: glucose, barley malt, maltose, molasses, cane juice crystals, lactose, corn sweetener, crystalline fructose, ethyl maltol, dextran, malt powder, fructose, maltodextrin, fruit juice concentrate, galactose, disaccharides, and dozens more.

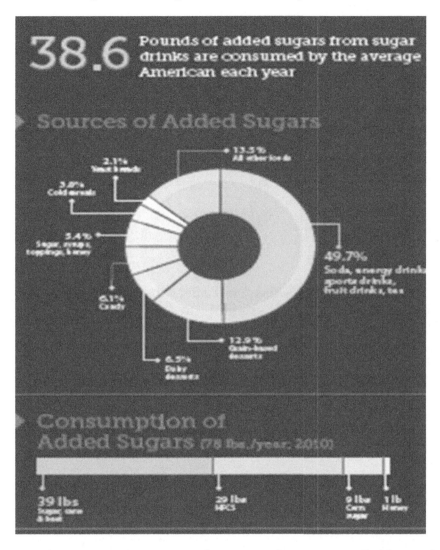

There are many types of processed sugars available, and they go by many names, so you may not recognize them all. The easiest way to avoid them is by not eating processed foods and eating whole foods instead.

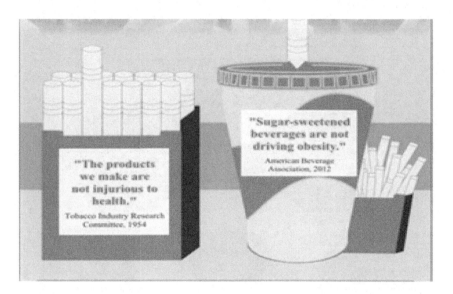

Eating sugar can negatively affect the hormone leptin by making your body resistant to its satiating effects. Consequently, your ability to get full after eating a sugary meal decreases due to leptin resistance. This means your body is producing it, but the brain is not responding to it, so you keep eating. The cycle that unfolds after eating sugar is one of the primary reasons that it causes weight gain.

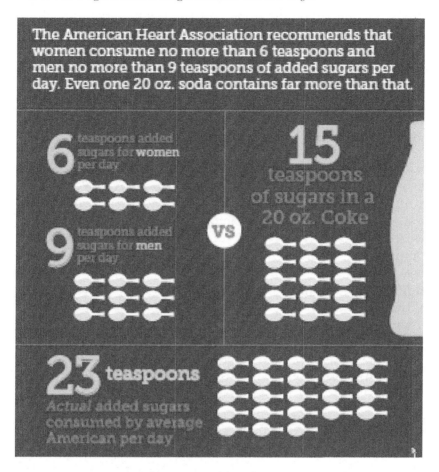

The American Heart Association recommends that women consume no more than 6 teaspoons and men no more than 9 teaspoons of added sugars per day. Even one 20 oz. soda contains far more than that.

6 teaspoons added sugars for **women** per day

9 teaspoons added sugars for **men** per day

VS

15 teaspoons of sugars in a 20 oz. Coke

23 teaspoons
Actual added sugars consumed by average American per day

68.   Avoid Artificial Sweeteners

Artificial sweeteners offer a sweet flavor and no calories. That's why people are attracted to drinking a sugar-free soda versus a sugar-sweetened soda with 150 calories. The most common artificial sweeteners are sucralose, saccharin, aspartame, acesulfame, and neotame.

One concern is that people who use artificial sweeteners sometimes eat more of other foods because they think they ate less by using artificial sweeteners.

Artificial sweeteners can alter the way we taste food by overstimulating our taste receptors since non-nutritive sweeteners can be up to 600 times sweeter than other sugars. They can damage your sugar receptors from frequent overstimulation and can limit tolerance for more sophisticated tastes causing people who use artificial sweeteners to find less intensely sweet foods, such as fruit, less appealing, and unsweet foods, such as vegetables, unpalatable. Synthetic sweeteners can cause you to avoid healthy foods and make you crave more artificially flavored foods with less nutritional value.

Artificial sweeteners may also prevent us from associating sweetness with caloric intake. So we end up wanting more sweets, choosing sweet food over nutritious food, and gaining weight. People who consume artificial sweeteners are twice as likely to become overweight compared to people who don't use them. Animal studies also show that artificial sweeteners can be twice as addictive as cocaine. Some synthetic sweeteners can also increase your risk of endocrine or hormone imbalances and cancer.

If you're craving something sweet, try foods that contain sugar naturally, such as fruit. Fruits are high in fiber, full of nutrients, and low in glycemic load.

69.   Decrease Salt Intake

People who eat more salt gain more weight for several reasons. First, eating salt increases the amount of sodium in your bloodstream. Excess salt upsets the balance of necessary sodium that has to be in your bloodstream and reduces your kidney's ability to remove the water. The excess fluid retained by your body, increases blood pressure and weight due to the extra water and additional strain on the delicate blood vessels leading to the kidneys.

Additionally, foods that tend to be higher in salt are also higher in calories, such as chips, snacks, fried foods, fast food, processed meats, and restaurant meals. Bread is the number one source of sodium in the Western diet. These foods are all high in sodium, carbohydrates, highly processed, chemicals, and notoriously easy to overeat.

Our brains and bodies are designed to crave salt because it's necessary for survival. Throughout human history, finding salt was difficult, so enjoying salt was a survival mechanism. Today, however, the average American overeats salt, and the more you consume, the more addictive it becomes.

Restaurants and processed food producers use salt to attract and retain customers by loading their foods with salt and using their addictive properties to maintain customers. Consuming foods high in salt increases your risk of obesity by 25%. Try using metabolism-boosting spices such as ginger, chili peppers, turmeric, cayenne, cinnamon, and mustard instead.

70. Garlic

The active ingredients in garlic are allicin, ajoene, allyl sulfides, and vinyldithiins. Garlic is also rich in vitamins B6 and C, fiber, calcium, protein, and manganese. Adding garlic into recipes is an easy way to boost energy levels, increase metabolism, burn fat efficiently, and detoxify your body. These qualities combine to boost your body's thermogenesis, suppress your appetite, and keep you fuller for longer, further preventing you from overeating. Add 1-2 teaspoons of garlic to your food a day for optimal results.

71. Ginger

Ginger contains chemicals called shogaols and gingerols. Gingerols help food digest faster, decrease inflammation, stabilize your blood sugar levels, and increase weight loss. Ginger makes you feel full, reducing hunger and increases thermogenesis, which burns more calories.

Ginger's antioxidant properties help prevent free radical damage that causes cardiovascular damage due to being overweight. Drink one cup a day of ginger tea or add one teaspoon of grated ginger to meals each day for optimal benefits.

72.   Black Pepper

Black pepper contains vitamins A, C, and K, minerals, fatty acids, and works as a natural metabolic booster. Pepper also contains a compound called piperine, which has fat burning and lipid-lowering properties that help you lose weight. Pepper has a thermogenic effect that increases your metabolic rate, so you burn calories hours after eating a meal. This thermogenic effect prevents the formation of new fat cells, suppresses fat accumulation, increases satiety, and helps you lose weight. Adding 1-2 peppercorns to each meal is enough to speed up your metabolism.

73.   Restock with Spices

Instead of using fatty dressing and sugary sauces, try healthy spices more often. Commercial food flavorings have chemicals that damage your endocrine system, add unnecessary calories to food, and cause weight gain. Spices are anti-inflammatory, increase metabolism, enhance fat burning, and promote feelings of fullness. Stocking your pantry with spices is an easy and effortless way to cut calories and increase weight loss.

74.   Saffron

Saffron is used to treat skin disease, respiratory issues, poor vision, pain, mental illness, erectile dysfunction, infections, and gynecological problems. It takes about 70,000 crocus flowers or 200,000 dried stigmas which are harvested by hand, to yield a pound of saffron. Due to the cultivation, harvesting, and handling, saffron can cost around $260 an ounce in the USA and is the most expensive spice in the world.

Saffron has over 150 chemicals in it, but the most studied are crocetin and crocin, picrocrocin, and safranal, which give saffron its color and odor. These compounds are all strong antioxidants, and they cause many of saffron's benefits.

Saffron is useful in the treatment of depression and

anxiety. Studies show that crocin, the active ingredient in saffron, is better at treating depression than Prozac, Zoloft, and Celexa, the most commonly used antidepressants. It also increases a person's mood, which helps cut down on snacking.

Saffron is effective in controlling compulsive eating by increasing brain levels of serotonin, which helps prevent compulsive overeating and the associated weight gain. As little as 1.5 grams of saffron a day can inhibit weight gain, block fat digestion, act as an antioxidant, decrease inflammation, suppress food intake by increasing satiety, and enhance glucose and lipid metabolism.

75.   Cinnamon

Cinnamon has multiple active ingredients, including cinnamaldehyde, eugenol, mucilage, tannins, carotenoids, and phenolics. Cinnamon boosts your metabolism because it takes more energy to digest than other foods. These ingredients help boost your metabolism, burn fat, decrease weight, and reduce fat deposited in the abdominal area. Cinnamon also helps reduce the absorption of fatty and high-calorie foods,

Cinnamon increases insulin sensitivity and lowers blood sugar, both important to controlling type 2 diabetes and heart disease.

Add one teaspoon to a fatty meal or a glass of warm water, half a lemons worth of juice, and honey for flavoring.

76.   Skip the Sea Salt

Sea salt has become very popular and often costs more than table salt, even though its nutritional content is similar to table salt. Table salt, on the other hand, has an advantage if you consume it iodized.

Your thyroid gland uses iodine to make thyroid hormones that help control growth, repair damaged cells, and support a healthy metabolism and weight. Being deficient in iodine can cause pregnancy-related issues, swelling in the neck, learning difficulties, and weight gain. Its symptoms are similar to those of hypothyroidism, or low thyroid hormones. Iodine deficiency is not common in the USA, but one-third of the world's population is deficient. Cooking with iodized salt is sufficient to help you meet your requirements.

77. Curry Leaves

Drinking tea made out of curry leaves can provide multiple health benefits, including; lowering cholesterol, regulating blood sugar, accelerating metabolism, improving digestion, detoxification, and weight loss.

Boil ten curry leaves in water for five minutes, strain the tea to remove the leaves and flavor with honey and lemon juice. Drink in the mornings on an empty stomach.

F. Fats

78. Eat More Fats

Dietary fat provides nutrients and helps with weight loss. Healthy fats help you feel satisfied, give food flavor, burn fat, balance hormone levels, decrease inflammation, boost cognitive performance, and are good for your health. Olive, coconut, avocado, and walnut oils, butter, and nut and seed butter (almond butter, peanut butter, and tahini) can help you slim down. For optimal weight loss, include some healthy fats with every meal and snack. For example, add nuts and oils to salads, nut butter to fruits, a fresh avocado as a side to your meat, and coconut oil-based mayonnaise to sandwiches.

79. Avocado Oil

Most cooking oils are made from fruits and vegetables, while avocado oil comes from the pulp of the fruit instead of the seeds.

That means you can eat many of the vitamins, minerals, and other nutrients of the avocado in a concentrated way. It's almost like eating an avocado.

Avocado oil has a high smoke point, which allows you to cook with it at high heat while preserving essential minerals, vitamins, and other nutrients. Avocado oil improves joint problems, digestion, vision, decreases cholesterol, fights cancer, and decreases aging. It's also great for salad. Using three tablespoons of avocado oil daily can help you lose two percent of your belly fat in a month.

80. Coconut Oil

Coconut oil is a type of fatty acid called a "medium-chain triglyceride." It works to decrease the accumulation of body fat and works as an appetite suppressant. This has a significant effect on increasing your metabolism, reducing hunger, boosting HDL (the "good") cholesterol, and helping you lose weight. Studies show that two tablespoons (30 ml) a day are enough to get the desired health benefits. Use coconut oil in place of other cooking oils, and add to coffee or tea.

81. MCT Oil

Medium-chain triglycerides (MCT) oil is extracted from coconut or palm kernel oil. MCT made from coconut is better quality and better for the environment as palm oil is grown on cleared rainforest land. MCT molecules are smaller than long-chain triglycerides (LCT), which is the triglyceride in most fats you eat, making them easier to digest. MCT is easy to absorb in your bloodstream, where it's quickly turned into energy you can use. MCT oil is separated from coconut or palm kernel oil and concentrated through a process called fractionation. Studies show MCT can be useful for weight loss, appetite control, extra energy for exercise, and decreasing inflammation. MCT oil has virtually no taste or smell, so it can be mixed into food or drinks without affecting the flavor.

82. Extra Virgin Olive Oil

As mentioned previously, vegetable oils (canola, corn, or soybean oils) are high in inflammatory omega-6 fatty acids, which can push your body into a state of chronic inflammation, causing weight gain and skin problems. Cold-pressed extra virgin olive oil is high in polyphenols, which lower blood pressure and oleic acid, which reduces appetite and promotes weight loss. Although olive oil has a moderate smoke point and can withstand being used for cooking, it is best served cold over salads or as a dip for bread.

Polyunsaturated oils should be consumed daily to ensure the regular production of eicosanoids. Eicosanoids are a powerful hormone that controls every cell, organ, and system in our body. These hormones control mounting or inhibiting inflammation, allergy, fever, and other immune responses, regulating normal childbirth, contributing to pain perception, regulating cell growth, controlling blood pressure, weight, and modulating blood to tissues' regional flow.

G. Beverages

83. Temperature of Beverages

Drink room temperature or warm water, not cold water. Your core temperature is 98.6 degrees Fahrenheit, while your refrigerator is 35 degrees. When you drink something that has a 60-degree difference, your body will slow digestion down to warm up the cold water. Not until it warms this water up does it get back to absorbing nutrients and burning fat.

84. Cranberry Juice

Unsweetened cranberry juice has a low glycemic index and is a low-calorie substitute for other beverages. It is also rich in antioxidants that help remove toxins from your body, fight infections, boost your metabolism, and decrease weight. Studies show that drinking a glass a day of cranberry juice can help reduce body mass index.

85. Parsley & Lemon Juice

Studies show that the combination of parsley and lemon juice can assist with weight loss. While lemon juice is a detoxifier, when combined with parsley, they can accelerate weight loss and help you lose belly fat.

Parsley contains vitamins A, B, C, and K as well as minerals such as iron and potassium. Parsley also helps maintain blood sugar levels, is a natural diuretic, flushes away toxins, and is a diuretic. The chlorophyll and enzymes improve digestion and promote weight loss. Lemon juice, hydrates, improves digestion and helps maintain the body's pH.

Parsley and lemon juice are high in vitamin C, which helps with digestion and fat oxidation for weight loss. Drink every morning for five days and then again after a break of 10 days. You can repeat as many times as desired, as both lemon and parsley are good for your general health.

86.   Lemon and Honey Water

The combination of lemon juice and honey has multiple health benefits, including weight loss. The vitamin C in the lemon helps oxidize fat, and the honey lowers lipid levels. Honey has numerous healing properties. It is an antibacterial, anti-inflammatory, and can heal wounds such as diabetic ulcers, and reduces coughing.

One lemon has an entire day's worth of vitamin C, a nutrient that reduces levels of cortisol, a stress hormone that triggers hunger and fat storage. Additionally, lemons contain polyphenols, which prevent fat accumulation and weight gain. Lemon peel has pectin, a soluble fiber that fills you up for longer. When possible, add whole blended lemons to your homemade smoothies or other beverages. Lemons contain nutrients and compounds that reduce the risk of chronic illnesses like heart disease, esophageal cancer, diabetes, and help prevent kidney stones.

First thing in the morning on an empty stomach, mix one teaspoon of honey and the juice from one lemon in a glass of warm water and drink.

Drinking honey lemon water can help you lose weight by increasing your metabolism and making you feel fuller. Drinking honey lemon water before meals will help reduce calorie intake.

87.   Coffee

If you drink decaffeinated coffee, you're missing out on a simple way to increase your metabolic burn temporarily. Caffeine stimulates your central nervous system and can increase your metabolism by 15% for up to 3 hours. One cup of coffee has 95 milligrams worth of caffeine and can increase your thermogenesis by up to 6%. Caffeine also has other health benefits such as lowered risk of cardiovascular disease, diabetes, and cognitive decline; decreased risk of premature death, and increased energy (especially as you age). As long as you don't have anxiety, acid reflux, heart disease, or other health concerns that are exacerbated by caffeine, then add caffeine to your diet.

If you drink coffee and have high cholesterol, use a paper filter. Unfiltered coffee (French press) contains cafestol, the most potent cholesterol-elevating substance known. Drinking four eight-ounce cups of French press coffee every day for four weeks could increase your cholesterol by 8 percent. Paper filters are the most effective at removing cafestol, single-serve options, like Keurig K-Cups, already have them built-in.

Avoid creamers. Two tablespoons of heavy cream adds 100 calories to your cup of coffee. If you drink two cups of coffee a day, not adding creamer to your coffee can add up to you losing 10 pounds in less than six months.

88.   Sweet Coffee Drinks

The caffeine in plain black coffee can boost your metabolism and increase fat burning. Sweetened coffee drinks are very high in calories (the same amount of calories as a meal), contain more sugar than soda, are loaded with artificial ingredients, and fattening. Although they do contain caffeine, the artificial cream and sugar outweigh the benefits. Adding small amounts of cream or milk is ok. Just avoid adding sugar, (low calorie sugar substitute or real sugar), high-calorie creamers, or other unhealthy ingredients. Drinking one of these coffees with a meal would be like eating two meals at once which can quickly increase your weight.

89.   Peppermint Tea

Peppermint tea helps with weight loss, reduces heartburn, makes your skin glow, induces sleep, and makes you feel full. It is excellent for boosting metabolism, decreasing acidity, clears acne when applied to the skin, aids in weight loss, suppresses appetite, and increases bile flow, which helps improve the digestion of fats. The most common method is to mix one handful of peppermint in a glass of warm water with lemon juice and a teaspoon of honey.

90. Cinnamon Tea

Drinking cinnamon tea decreases blood sugar due to cinnamon's effect on blood glucose. Cinnamon tea has multiple health benefits. It boosts your metabolism, keeps your cholesterol and blood sugar level in check, and is anti-inflammatory to help prevent bloating. It also aids in digestion which helps control weight as well. There are several ways to prepare cinnamon tea. The most common method is to mix one teaspoon of cinnamon in a glass of warm water with lemon juice and a teaspoon of honey.

91. Green Tea

Studies show that drinking 2 and 3 cups of green tea throughout the day will help you lose around one pound per month or 100 calories over 24 hours, even if you stick to your regular diet. Green tea is rich in epigallocatechin and gallic acid (EGCG), a type of catechin and caffeine; both play a significant role in weight loss. EGCG is a potent antioxidant, and caffeine burns calories. Although not as effective as a cup of green tea, taking green tea extract (50 mg caffeine and 90 mg EGCG) with each meal burns 4% more calories over 24 hours.

92. Oolong Tea

Oolong tea combines some of the good qualities of both black and green teas. It is made from the leaves of the same plants used to make green and black tea. The difference is in how long the leaves are allowed to oxidize. All tea leaves contain enzymes that oxidize them. Green tea is allowed to oxidize very little, then oolong tea, and then black tea is a green tea that is allowed to oxidize until it turns black.

Oolong tea has antioxidants known as tea polyphenols (theaflavins, thearubigins, and EGCG). It's also rich in theanine, an amino acid responsible for the tea's calming effect.

Oolong tea accelerates your metabolism, improves fat mobilization, prevents fat cell growth, helps promote weight loss, and builds immunity as it is loaded with more antioxidants than green tea. For optimal benefits drink oolong tea three times a day.

93. White Tea

White tea is high in caffeine, antioxidants, and catechins like EGCG. These compounds work synergistically to burn fat and boost your metabolism. White tea is produced from the same plant as green, oolong, and black tea but is less processed, which makes it higher in antioxidants and gives it a unique flavor. White tea reduces the risk of heart disease, Alzheimer's and Parkinson's diseases, diabetes, inflammation, skin aging, colon cancer, osteoporosis, and helps with weight loss.

White tea has a plant-based antioxidant called polyphenols. Antioxidants protect the cells from damage to the body caused by free radicals. Polyphenols like those found in white tea help reduce the risk of heart disease, boost immunity, burn fat, and boost your metabolism by an extra 4–5% (burning an additional 70–100 calories per day).

White tea also has fluoride, catechins, and tannins. This combination of compounds helps strengthen teeth, fight bacteria and sugar, and prevent cavities. Also, white tea lowers the risk of insulin resistance and improves blood sugar control for increased weight loss. Two to three cups a day of white tea will give you the desired health effects.

94. Pu-erh Tea

Pu-erh tea is a type of fermented black tea. It comes from the same tea leaves used for green, oolong, and black tea. Studies show that Pu-erh tea can lower blood sugar, blood triglycerides, suppresses appetite, and increase weight loss. Drinking 2-3 cups a day can help you lose approximately 0.7 pounds a month.

69

95.   Herbal Teas

Herbal teas are a mixture of herbs, spices, or fruit in hot water. They're different from other teas because they don't usually contain caffeine or traditional tea leaves. The most common herbal teas include rooibos tea, ginger tea, hibiscus tea, and rosehip tea. Herbal teas have antioxidants, help you feel satiated, burn fat, control blood sugar, promote weight loss, increase fat metabolism, and help block the formation of fat cells. Drink 2-3 cups a day to achieve the mentioned benefits.

96.   Cook with Tea

If you're not fond of tea or want more of its fat-burning properties in your diet, try using it for cooking. When you're making vegetable soup, beans, rice, oatmeal, or any other dish that requires water, use brewed tea in your recipes instead.

97.   Sugary Drinks

One of the easiest ways to cut calories is to limit products that have added sugar. Sugar-sweetened drinks, like sugary coffees, iced teas, and soda are some of the unhealthiest foods ever created. Not only do they cause significant weight gain, but they can cause multiple adverse health effects even in low quantities. The danger with soft drinks is that even though they have a lot of calories, your brain doesn't register them like solid food. So you can drink a full meal's worth of calories and still not feel full. Sugar in liquid form (a can of soda has around 9.5 tsp of sugar per 12 ounces) won't make you feel full, so you'll keep eating. Instead, you end up adding the calories from your beverage on top of whatever you eat. Sugary drinks also promote fat storage around your midsection. If you can't cut them out of   your   diet,   then   consume   smaller   portions.

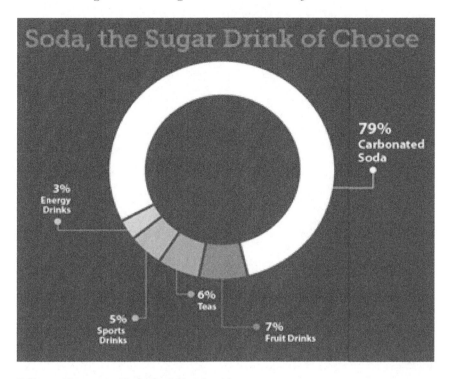

98. Sugary Drink Alternatives

Regular consumption of artificially sweetened and sugary drinks is linked to increased body fat. A glass of water with ginger, lemon, herbs, or fruit will help curb cravings for sugary drinks and keep you hydrated.

Other alternatives to soft drinks include water with fresh mint, ginger, berries, cucumber, lime, or lemon. Herbal, green, and black teas are another option and come with additional health benefits. Unsweetened seltzer or flavored carbonated water is especially effective because it fills your stomach with gas making you feel full. Trimming calories from liquid drinks will help you lose more weight than cutting solid foods.

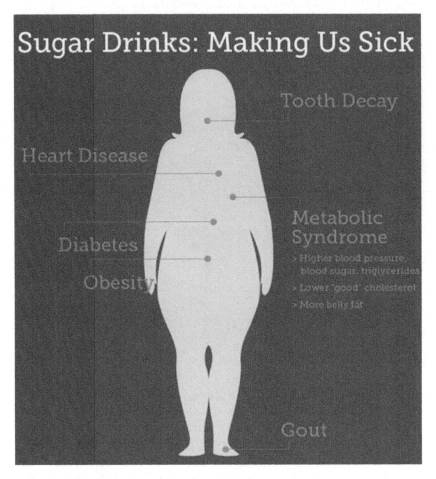

Sugar Drinks: Making Us Sick

Tooth Decay

Heart Disease

Metabolic Syndrome
> Higher blood pressure, blood sugar, triglycerides
> Lower 'good' cholesterol
> More belly fat

Diabetes

Obesity

Gout

99.   Blending Versus Juicing

Juicing fruits and vegetables removes all the fiber, leaving only the liquid. Blending keeps all of the pulp and fiber from the produce. Juicing has the advantage of concentrating vitamins and nutrients and easier absorption of nutrients. However, some juices have more sugar than sodas, and you lose valuable fiber. Fiber is vital for healthy digestion, weight management, decreasing your risk of heart disease, and controlling blood sugar.

If you love juice, try blending your fruits and vegetables with water. Blending keeps all the fiber for digestion, improves weight management, retains all nutrients (not as concentrated as juice), and contains multiple phytonutrient compounds. Although the pulp in blended drinks may be unappetizing to some, you'll consume much less and stay full longer, leading to more significant weight loss.

100. Add Fiber to Drinks

Fiber helps decrease appetite, and by suppressing your appetite, you're more likely to reduce your caloric intake, which can help you lose weight.

When you make homemade smoothies, add chunks of fruit, oats, wheat germ, or ground flaxseed. Adding fiber to your drinks and meals will counteract your body's tendency to store fat around the midsection. Whole grains and fibers have been proven to lower your body mass index.

101. Forgetting to Drink Water for Extended Periods

Not drinking water for long lengths of time during the day can cause weight gain.

Your metabolism is a sum of all of your bodily functions that use energy: thinking, digestion, muscle contraction, elimination of bodily waste, etc. Water plays a role in all body functions. When you're dehydrated, all of those processes will work in a less efficient manner, which could slow down your metabolism. An excellent way to remember to drink enough water each day is to use a visual reminder such as keeping a reusable bottle close by to remind you to keep drinking.

Drinking half a liter (17 ounces) water approximately 30 minutes before a meal can help you eat less and lose weight. Over a 12-week period, you can lose 44% more weight compared to people who do not drink water before a meal. If you're replacing sugary drinks with water, you'll experience an even greater effect.

Dehydration can make you think you're hungry. To prevent this, drink at least eight ounces of water every hour. The body craves sweets when it lacks water.

102. Increase Water Intake

Drinking eight glasses of water a day is the general recommendation. However, a more precise amount depends on your weight, activity level, and the environment where you live. For optimal health, drink between half an ounce to one ounce of water for each pound of body weight every day. For example, if you weigh 200 pounds, you should drink between 100-200 ounces (12.5-25 glasses) of water a day. If you exercise regularly or live in a hot climate, you're going to be on the higher end of that recommendation; if you live in colder weather and mostly sedentary, you'd need much less.

To assist with digestion and decrease hunger, drink one glass of water 30 minutes before a meal. Wait at least an hour after the meal to drink water to allow the body to absorb the nutrients.

Sixty percent of the time when we think we're hungry, we're actually thirsty and we inappropriately respond to thirst by eating instead of drinking. The same part of your brain controls hunger and thirst, and sometimes it mixes up the signals. Keeping a water bottle around will help you respond to thirst correctly.

Staying well hydrated helps your body stop retaining water, causing you to shed extra pounds of water weight. Drinking water before a meal, approximately 500 ml (a little over 2 cups) thirty minutes before a meal, will cause you to eat 13% fewer calories per meal. People who drink at least 1.53 liters of water a day, after their coffee, juice, milk, or whatever else they drink will cause them to consume an average of 193 fewer (or 9%) calories a day. Adding lemon, orange, lime, sliced cucumber, or berries to water will give it a good flavor. Filter your water at home and transport it in your glass or metal containers to avoid harmful chemicals associated with plastic bottles.

Best time to drink water.

1. When you wake up, consume two to three cups of water

to help you wake up naturally without coffee and cleanse the body.

2. To decrease hunger, drink a glass of water half an hour before a meal.

3. Drink a glass of water to help wash down a meal at least an hour after a meal.

4. When you feel tired, drink a glass of water instead of a cup of coffee.

5. Instead of taking aspirin, drink water when you have a headache.

6. Drink water before, during, and after exercise.

7. Take a drink or two of water before bedtime and keep an extra-large container next to your bed so that you can drink it first thing in the morning.

103. The Best Water to Drink

The best water to drink is water that is not bottled or packaged. Water that has been packaged in plastic bottles is toxic as it contains residue and chemicals from plastic. One of them is phthalates, or phthalate esters, which are esters of phthalic acid. They are mainly added to plastics to increase their flexibility, transparency, durability, and longevity. The second most common is bisphenol A (BPA), an industrial chemical used to make plastics. Both substances have been found to cause several types of cancers, unbalance your endocrine system, and damage to fetuses. Your best option will be to use a reverse osmosis (RO) machine ($150) to filter your water. It can filter particles as small as 0.001 microns. The second, and much more economical option, is an activated carbon water filter, such as a Brita water filter ($12). Activated-carbon filters are rated by the size of the particles they can remove, and generally range from 50 microns (least effective) to 0.5 microns (most effective). Most toxic microplastics are about 2.5 micrometers in size. Either way, use refillable glass or metal containers to carry and drink your water from to avoid consuming some of these dangerous chemicals associated with plastic bottles.

104. Drink Water as Soon as You Get Up

Optimal hydration is vital to helping your body function at its peak performance. Insufficient hydration of even 2%, can cause fatigue and cloudy thinking.

Water is essential to every cell in your body. For example, lung tissue is made up of nearly 90% water. Your blood is more than 80% water. And, your brain is approximately 70% water.

Most people wake up dehydrated after not drinking water throughout the night and losing moisture with every breath while sleeping. Drinking water first thing in the morning is an excellent way to increase alertness, rehydrate, aid digestion, decrease hunger, improve mental acuity, and lower your insulin levels. Since you've been without eating for an average of eight hours, your body will want calories, so insulin levels are highest when you wake up each morning, meaning that whatever you eat is going to be stored at a higher percentage resulting in increased fat storage. Drinking water helps decrease your insulin levels, reduce hunger, and decrease weight gain. Studies show that people who drink two glasses (16 ounces) of water before their first meal can lose, on average, one pound per month.

Drink three to four glasses when you wake up every morning to rehydrate your body quickly. Add a dash of ocean salt or pink salt to help balance electrolytes and some fresh pressed lemon juice to make the water alkaline and lower your body's acidity. Many of the body's processes produce acid, leading to multiple health issues and causing weight gain. Drinking lemon water will reduce the acidity in your body and make you more alkaline. Having your body's pH in the optimal range helps facilitate weight loss.

Ten Benefits of Drinking Water First Thing in the

Morning.

1. It helps you move your lower bowels for regularity in the mornings.

2. Water increases your level of alertness. It can have the same effect as coffee or tea, except that it won't cause further dehydration like coffee and tea due to their caffeine content.

Water will also stimulate faster growth of red blood cells in your system and generates more oxygen in your blood, which will boost your energy.

3. Boosts your brain capacity. Your brain is made up of over 70% water and keeping it well hydrated will increase optimal brain activity. Not having enough water can cause fatigue, mood fluctuations, decreased memory, and reduced brain performance.

4. Strengthens your immune system.

5. Clear's toxins produced during the nightly bodily repairs performed during sleep.

6. Boosts your metabolic rate for the rest of the day helping maintain an ideal body weight.

7. Promotes weight loss by helping you feel satiated, reducing your cravings for the day, and reducing overeating.

8. Releases toxins from your body, which improves skin complexion and radiance.

9. Water keeps your body hydrated, which is vital for the proper functioning of internal organs. Drinking water first thing in the morning prevents kidney stones and protects your colon and bladder from infections.

10. Staying hydrated will make your hair glow and keep your bones full of the water they need to grow correctly.

105. Fruit Juices

Fruit juices are high in calories, often have added sugar, and usually contain no fiber. Eating whole fruit is always a healthier option. In fact, most fruit juices have very little in common with whole fruit. Fruit juices are usually highly processed, pasteurized, and loaded with sugar. All of this processing removes many of the health benefits that are typically found in the whole fruit. Fruit juice usually ends up having as much sugar and calories as soda, if not more. Due to the lack of fiber, a glass of orange juice won't make you feel as full as if you ate the fruit itself, making it easy to consume large quantities in a short amount of time. Avoid fruit juice and eat whole fruit instead.

106. Cold-pressed Juice

Cold-pressed juice preserves the nutrients of the fruits and vegetables from heat. The heat from electric juicers can diminish the nutrients in the juice. Since cold press juicers use manpower to extract the juice, no heat is involved. That means your juice will have a higher nutrient content, which can improve health and boost weight loss.

However, juices are high in sugar and calories, even if they're cold-pressed. Drinking fresh fruit juice can contribute to excess calorie consumption, which may cause you to gain weight. Make juices that contain low-sugar veggies like celery and fruits like lemon to control your calorie intake.

107. Coconut Water

Coconut water is a popular natural beverage and is excellent for use as an electrolyte. However, even though coconut water has minerals, vitamins, and antioxidants, it does have sugar and calories. One 8 oz. cup (240 ml) of coconut water has 6 grams of sugar and 45 calories. Coconut water is also a juice, and even though it is lower in sugar and calories than soda and other juices, it's best to limit your consumption of any sweet beverage.

108. The Effects of Alcohol on Weight Loss

- **Alcohol Affects the Absorption of Nutrients and Digestion**

All types of alcohol can impair digestion and absorption of nutrients.

Alcohol can stress the stomach and the intestines, which decreases digestive secretions and movement of food through the intestinal tract.

Digestive secretions are essential to breaking down food into micro- and macronutrients that are absorbed into the body. Not absorbing nutrients completely will cause difficulties with managing your weight.

- **Alcohol Contains Empty Calories**

Alcoholic beverages provide your body with calories but not nutrients. A 12-ounce can of beer contains 155 calories, and a 5-ounce glass of red wine has 125 calories. Mixed drinks, made with fruit juice or soft drinks, can be even higher in calories. By comparison, a donut has 190 calories. Therefore a night out with several drinks can easily lead to consuming a few hundred to over a thousand extra calories.

- **Alcohol is Burned as a Primary Fuel**

Besides calorie content, when you drink alcohol, your body burns it as a primary fuel source before anything else. Excess glucose and lipids in your diet are burned after the alcohol and often end up being stored as fat.

- **Alcohol Affects Hormones**

Alcohol can lower your testosterone levels. Testosterone is a sex hormone that is critical in many metabolic processes, including fat burning and muscle formation. Having low testosterone can cause multiple health problems including:

- o high cholesterol
- o high blood pressure
- o difficulty sleeping
- o high blood sugar levels
- o high body mass index

- **Alcohol Can Affect Fat Metabolism**

The liver is the body's filter, it filters the blood and removes foreign substances, including drugs and alcohol. The liver also helps in the metabolism of proteins, fats, and carbohydrates.

Drinking too much alcohol can cause alcoholic fatty liver. Damage to your liver will affect the way your body metabolizes and stores fats and carbohydrates. This condition will change the way your body stores energy from food and make it difficult to lose weight.

- **Alcohol Can Cause Sleeplessness**

Alcohol can disturb your sleep cycles and cause sleeplessness. Sleep deprivation, from lack of sleep or impaired sleep, can imbalance your hormones which can affect your feelings of hunger, satiety, and cause weight gain.

- **Alcohol Can Cause Excess Belly Fat**

Foods high in simple sugars, such as beer, candy, and soda, are high in calories. Alcohol speeds up the process of digestion, which breaks down glucose rapidly, and causes insulin to grab glucose and store it away. Extra calories are not burned up and end up stored as body fat. This process causes a beer gut as the abdominal area tends to accumulate fat.

- **Alcohol Affects Food Choices**

Alcohol lowers inhibitions, leading to poor food choices, and can trigger hunger signals in the brain, increasing the urge to eat more food.

109. Five Best Alcoholic Beverages for Weight Loss

Drinking in moderation will help you enjoy a healthier body, sleep better, and improve digestion. If you're going to drink there are alternative ways to drink and still lose weight.

- **Brandy**

Brandy is best served as an after-dinner digestive aid.

100 calories per 1.5 ounces of brandy

- **Vodka**

Mix with low-calorie mixers (club soda) and avoid juices high in sugar.

100 calories per 1.5 ounces of distilled 80-proof vodka

- **Whiskey**

Don't mix with soft drinks, but instead drink on the rocks.

100 calories per 1.5 ounces of 86-proof whiskey

- **Tequila**

Drink tequila in the customary shot glass with just salt, lime, and tequila.

100 calories per 1.5 ounces of tequila

- **Gin**

Drink gin in a martini with olives.

115 calories per 1.5 ounces of 90-proof gin.

110. If You're Going to Drink, Do So After Dinner

Eating out can ruin your hard-earned weight loss, and

so can drinking alcohol. To help you reach your ideal weight goals, order your cocktail or glass of wine at the end of your meal. The sweet sugars in the alcohol can help you feel satiated and can act as a low-cal dessert. Plus, drinking before a meal lowers your inhibition and can cause you to order something unhealthy off the menu.

H. Dairy Products

Milk and other dairy products are the top sources of saturated fat in the American diet, contributing to type 2 diabetes, heart disease, and Alzheimer's. Studies have linked dairy to an increased risk of ovarian, breast, and prostate cancers. Dairy products are liquid meat, high fat, high cholesterol with no dietary fiber. Dairy products are generally not good for you. They're high in artificial hormones and bovine hormones which help calves get fat and large quickly.

The chemicals in cheese can be as addictive as heroin. Studies show that the higher the intake of calcium, the higher the rate of osteoporosis. For example, Japan has one of the lowest rates of osteoporosis due largely to the nonconsumption of dairy products. Whereas the United States has one of the highest rates of osteoporosis in the world due to the large consumption of dairy products.

If you prefer to keep dairy products in your diet the following are some healthy alternatives.

111. Frozen Yogurt

Because frozen yogurt is considered a healthier alternative to ice cream, it's frequently over-consumed. Many frozen yogurt shops allow you to self-serve your desert, making portion control difficult. To keep your intake under control, pick the smallest yogurt cup available. Additionally, the sugary toppings offered at most frozen yogurt shops can add even more calories and sugar. Choose natural toppings like fresh fruit (avoid canned fruits in syrup), unsweetened coconut, and nuts (especially walnuts for their high levels of brain-healthy omega-3 fatty acids). Also, avoid non-fat and sugar-free yogurts to avoid all the chemicals that are associated with weight gain. Lastly, avoid waffle bowls, syrups, and sauces.

112. Ice Cream

Commercially made ice cream is high in sugar and very unhealthy. It is high in calories, artificial colors, and loaded with sugar. Consider sherbet, healthy low-fat, or homemade ice cream which contains less sugar and healthier ingredients such as greek yogurt and fruit. Just be mindful of portions so that you don't overeat.

113. Kefir

Kefir, on average, has twice as much protein as yogurt. It can also have up to 61 strains of bacteria compared to the 2-3 in yogurt. Due to the high content of probiotics, kefir is usually lactose-free. Different kinds of milk, including nut or dairy, are used to make kefir. Kefir prevents cancer, detoxifies the body, improves intestinal health, and promotes weight loss. The high protein content helps keep you satiated, and the good bacteria helps keep your gut healthy for optimal digestion.

Cheese

114. Parmesan

Parmesan cheese is high in protein, and has more calcium than any other cheese. These two attributes help control sugar, sugar cravings, and help the body metabolize fat. Foods that are high in protein and calcium such as Parmesan cheese increase the body's core temperature, which increases thermogenesis, and thus boosts your metabolism. It's also a low-lactose food, so those who are lactose intolerant can eat it.

The Italian cheese also has the amino acid tyrosine which stimulates the brain to release dopamine without any unhealthy insulin spikes. It also has approximately 2 grams of protein, and only 12 calories and 1 gram of fat per tablespoon. Another good thing about parmesan is that a small amount has a lot of taste and packs the same amount of calcium, protein, and minerals as other cheeses. It's great as a replacement for high calories cheeses in pasta dishes. Also, opt for better quality parmesan as the lower quality ones are mixed with wood sawdust (cellulose) to cut down on costs. Cellulose is not necessarily bad for you, but it reduces the benefits of the cheese.

115. Feta

Feta is low in calories, fat, and is a staple in the heart-healthy Mediterranean diet. It's potent flavor goes a long way with just a small amount. It's also high in calcium, protein, B vitamins, phosphorus, beneficial bacteria, and fatty acids. Feta is a good source of the amino acid histidine, which is vital to the conversion of protein into muscle. However, it is high in sodium. One ounce of feta cheese has 316 mg of sodium, 75 calories, 6 grams of fat, and 4 grams of protein.

116. Cheddar

Cheddar cheese is a lower-calorie, versatile cheese that can add a lot of flavor to many meals. One slice or about 1 ounce of cheddar cheese has about 113 calories, vitamins A, B2, and B12, calcium, magnesium, phosphorus, 7 grams of protein, and zinc.

117. Low-fat Cottage Cheese (1% to 2% Milkfat)

Cottage cheese is high in protein, low fat, high in B vitamins, calcium, phosphorus, and selenium. In particular, cottage cheese has casein protein, which is slowly absorbed, promotes muscle gain, and helps prevent muscle breakdown. Cottage cheese can help reduce the risk of developing insulin resistance, heart disease, improve bone health, and provide antioxidant protection. One cup of low cottage cheese provides 163 calories, 2.3 grams of fat, and 28 grams of protein.

118. Swiss

Swiss cheese has a bacterium called propionibacterium

freudenreichii, which reduces inflammation, slows the aging process, and boosts the immune system. Swiss cheese is also high in vitamin B12 (14% of RDI), calcium, phosphorus, and magnesium. One slice of swiss cheese has approximately 106 calories, 8 grams, and 7.5 grams of protein.

119. Goat Cheese

Goat cheese is a hypoallergenic alternative to cheese made with cow's milk. Goat milk has more calcium, potassium, and vitamin A than cow's milk, but cow's milk has more vitamin B12, selenium, and folic acid.

Goat cheese is also high in medium-chain fatty acids that can improve satiety and benefit weight loss.

A one-ounce (28-gram) serving of soft-style goat cheese has approximately 102 calories, 8 grams of fat, and 6 grams of protein.

Cheeses to Avoid

120. Cheese Sauce

Some cheese sauces have no real cheese at all and are made entirely of chemicals. It's best to eat real cheese and avoid the blowback from eating all the chemicals in nacho cheese sauce.

121. Cream Cheese

One tablespoon of cream cheese has 46 calories from fat, a small amount of carbs, one gram of protein, riboflavin (vitamin B2), and vitamin A. Try whipped cream cheese for a lighter, reduced-fat option.

122. American Cheese

American cheese is a "cheese product" or a "cheese snack." It isn't considered cheese because it doesn't contain at least 51% real cheese. That is why the label reads "pasteurized prepared cheese product." American cheese is made up mostly of processed ingredients, including vegetable oils and food dyes that give it it's unnatural yellow-orange color. Because of all the additives, it can last up to a year. American cheese is considered one of the worst cheeses for your health. One slice of American cheese has over 300 milligrams of sodium, which can cause weight gain, high blood pressure, hypertension, and heart disease. One slice of American cheese contains 10 grams of fat and 5 grams of protein.

123. Yogurt

People who eat three cups of yogurt a day will lose 22% more weight and 61% more body fat than people who only cut calories. Eating foods rich in probiotics boosts your metabolism and helps you lose more weight.

Eating calcium and protein-rich foods together magnifies their weight-loss ability. When combined, these two nutrient groups have been clinically proven to raise metabolism and improve digestion and bowel health.

Flavored yogurt is filled with artificial sweeteners and added sugar. An eight-ounce serving can have more than 30 grams of sugar. Flavor your plain yogurt with chopped fruit instead of buying it pre-mixed.

124. Pick 2% Over the Non-Fat Dairy

People who eat full-fat dairy tend to weigh less and gain less weight over time than those who consume non-fat products. Non-fat foods are less filling due to their low-fat content. Besides, they are often made with artificial ingredients and added sugar to give them flavor due to the lack of fat. Foods that contain fat digest slower, so they make you feel satiated longer and help you lose weight.

I. Exposure to Light

125. Near-Infrared Light (NIR) Therapy

Near-infrared light (NIR) therapy is a scientifically proven modality used for treating some of the common underlying ailments that lead to obesity, such as pain and depression. NIR light is a specific wavelength of light that donates photons to your mitochondria via molecules called cytochromes, promoting cell repair, decreasing pain and inflammation, promoting weight loss, and enhancing the healing process.

Its ability to penetrate deep down into the skin allows it to reach the cells' mitochondria, also known as the cell's power plants, and stimulate them to increase adenosine triphosphate (ATP) production. Resulting in recharging of your mitochondria, stimulation of DNA and RNA synthesis, increased blood flow, which activates the lymphatic system, resulting in increased waste removal and tissue repair. Increased ATP provides you with steady energy all day and better sleep at night. Red light also triggers collagen synthesis, and collagen represents more than 90% of the bone and 80% of the skin matrix. More collagen also means younger-looking skin and faster wound healing.

Different hues of light have various therapeutic effects on the body.

Red light stimulates melatonin production, which will help you improve your sleep and promote recovery during sleep. If used a few minutes before physical exercise, red and infrared light can boost strength and prevent soreness. Wavelengths of red and infrared light 660 to 905 nanometers reach skeletal muscle tissue, stimulating the mitochondria to produce more ATP, which cells use as fuel.

Although excessive exposure to blue light from electronics at night can be detrimental, exposure to blue light during the day can improve reaction time, alertness, focus, and productivity. High amounts of bright daylight hitting photoreceptors in the eye will suppress melatonin levels and set off receptors in the brain that energize you. Stand or sit by windows or go outside as much as possible every day to increase your dosage of blue rays from natural light.

Green light can reduce chronic pain caused by migraines or fibromyalgia by up to 60 percent. Green light increases the production of pain-killing opioid-like chemicals called enkephalins. Enkephalins reduce inflammation, which plays a role in many chronic pain conditions. One to two hours of green light a day can decrease migraines and other types of chronic pain.

126. Full-Spectrum Light

As a kid, I used full-spectrum light to help my pet reptiles stay healthy and produce vitamin D. If you have limited mobility or live somewhere with limited sunlight. A sun lamp or tanning bed high in UVB waves will give you many of the benefits of sunlight. UVB (as opposed to other ultraviolet rays) causes less tissue damage and offers more benefits. Tanning with UVB increases melanin in the skin, which acts as a sunscreen, increases vitamin D production, decreases inflammation, and can help eliminate skin issues like psoriasis, vitiligo, atopic dermatitis, and localized scleroderma.

Use a full-spectrum light, UVB lamp, or UVB-heavy tanning bed with a wavelength of 311-313 nanometers for 5 minutes, twice a week, to get more benefits than taking a vitamin D supplement. UVA is responsible for sunburn and skin aging, so avoid exposing your face and neck to prevent wrinkles.

UV exposure will also increase nitric oxide (NO), which reduces blood pressure, improves cardiovascular health, improves mood through the release of endorphins, and increases weight loss.

127. Avoid Blue Light at Night

White light from sunlight is a spectrum of the colors red, orange, yellow, green, blue, indigo, and violet. When that white light hits water drops in the atmosphere after rain, it scatters or gets separated, and we see a rainbow. Sunlight is also the primary source of blue light, which is what makes the sky look blue. Being outdoors during daylight will expose you to large doses of it.

There are also many artificial indoor sources of blue light, such as display screens of computers, electronic notebooks, smartphones, compact light (CFL) fluorescent and light-emitting diode (LED) lighting, and flat-screen televisions. Researchers have found no matter what you eat, exposure to artificial light leads to weight gain. Switch out the CFL and LED lights in your bedroom for incandescent, halogen, or at least soft white light bulbs.

Electronics emit only a fraction of the blue light produced by the sun, however, the average person is spending a lot of time using these devices, and the proximity of these screens to the user's face is causing multiple eye health problems. Blue light exposure at night can cause weight gain, cancer, diabetes, and heart disease. It also disrupts your sleep quality and duration, which can disrupt hormones, cause inflammation, mitochondrial dysfunction, increase food consumption, and result in reduced physical activity.

Read a book two to three hours before bedtime and avoid screen time. If you work at night or use a lot of electronics at night, wear blue-blocking glasses or use an app that filters the blue/green wavelength at night. Most smartphones have a feature in their setting for a night light or blue light filter. If you use night lights, use dim red lights, which have the least power to shift circadian rhythm and suppress melatonin. Get lots of natural sunlight during the day, which will help regulate hormone levels, improve sleep at night, mood, and performance during.

128. Cut Exposure to Light While You're Asleep

Exposure to light at night from streetlights, night lights,

lights from electronics, or the glare of a bedroom TV can disrupt sleep and circadian rhythms. Light helps regulate circadian rhythm, the body's internal clock that signals when to rest and when to be alert. Light also affects the production of the essential sleep-promoting hormone melatonin. Light exposure before or during bedtime can make it difficult to fall and stay asleep because your brain won't make enough sleep-inducing melatonin. Even if you're able to fall asleep with lights on in your bedroom, you may not get enough rapid eye movement (REM) sleep. REM sleep is the most essential of all for feeling rested and staying healthy.

Exposure to light at night disrupts sleep, alters eating behaviors, and can promote weight gain. Women who sleep in dark bedrooms are 21% less likely to be obese than those sleeping in rooms with light. Reduce exposure to artificial light at night using blackout shades, place dark tape over light sources on electronics, and remove all other light-emitting sources.

129. Open the Curtains

When you wake up in the mornings, open the curtains and let the sunlight in to help synchronize your circadian rhythms. Studies show that exposing yourself to sunlight for at least 45 minutes in the mornings between 6 and 9 am, increases your metabolism, burns fat, reduces appetite, and accelerates weight loss.

130. Get Morning Sun

Being exposed to direct sunlight between 8 a.m. and noon reduces your risk of weight gain despite your age, level of activity, or caloric intake. Sunlight undercuts your fat-storage genes and synchronizes your metabolism. A spectrum of the sun called blue-light can penetrate the skin and decrease the size of subdermal fat cells. In other words, it helps with fat loss, synchronizes your metabolism, and undercuts your fat-storage genes.

131. Use Sunlight as a Nutritional Supplement

Sunlight is vital for all animals, although some need different amounts and in different ways. Humans need sunlight to increase the production of essential nutrients such as;

Vitamin D

Vitamin D a hormone the kidneys produce that controls blood calcium concentration, multiple reactions in the body, and impacts the immune system.

Testosterone

Testosterone influences mental health, sex drive, muscle tone, and body composition. Direct sunlight on your chest and back can increase testosterone in men by 120%, and sunlight on your testicles can increase production by 200-400%.

Cholesterol Sulfate

Your body uses cholesterol sulfate to make all of your sex hormones.

Nitric Oxide

Nitric oxide (NO) causes vasodilation, increasing blood flow, oxygen, and nutrient transport through your body, and removing cellular waste. The increased blood flow also prevents heart attacks, improves athletic performance, recovery, lowers your blood pressure, and decreases inflammation.

Endorphins and Dopamine

These hormones help you relax, reduce pain, boost mood, inhibit cancer growth, and support hormone regulation.

132. Work Outdoors

To help remediate the negative impact of artificial light, work by a window or outside. People who get more sunlight are healthier, sleep better (46 minutes more sleep per night), and have fewer problems sleeping than those who don't. Not getting at least 30 minutes a day of sunlight is the equivalent to smoking a pack of cigarettes each day. Increasing exposure to sunlight intensifies motivation to exercise, boosts weight loss, and improves overall health. Sunlight kick-starts the fat-burning of brown adipose tissue in the body. As the fat burns, it transfers energy into heat, which boosts calorie burning.

J. Water

133. Use a Sauna

Use a sauna three times a week, up to twenty minutes at a time to release toxins from your liver, fat tissue, loosen joints, reduce stiffness, increase circulation, and burn calories. During a sauna session, core temperatures increase, the body cools itself down, causing a beneficial sweat. The heat created by a sauna does not directly produce significant amounts of weight loss, however, the sweating process helps eliminate heavy metals and toxic chemicals. The skin is your largest organ, and removing toxins through the skin, relieves the burden on the kidneys and liver and allows your body to function more efficiently and indirectly aids in weight loss.

134. Hang Out in a Tub

Water offers unparalleled health benefits. It strengthens muscles, ligaments, and improves your cardiovascular fitness. Due to buoyancy, it provides a safe and effective workout while gently supporting your body, particularly if you have injuries.

Because water creates a thermal effect of sucking heat away from your body, your body must burn more calories to maintain core body temperature. Water is 24 times more thermally conductive than air. That's why you can burn up to 24 times more energy in the water than you normally would outside of water. Think about the times you've been to the beach. Do you remember how hungry you felt afterward? That hunger was due to the caloric deficit you formed while being in the water. If you hang out in room temperature water for an hour without swimming, you'll burn twice as many calories as if you had gone jogging for an hour. The colder the water, the more time you spend in the water, and the more activity you engage in water, the more calories you'll burn. So you can sit in the bathtub or pool reading the paper while your body burns calories and you lose weight.

Water activities also put less pressure on the body; the buoyancy of the water helps support your body weight, taking the pressure off joints. Depending on how much you immerse your body into the water will determine how much weight you put on your extremities.

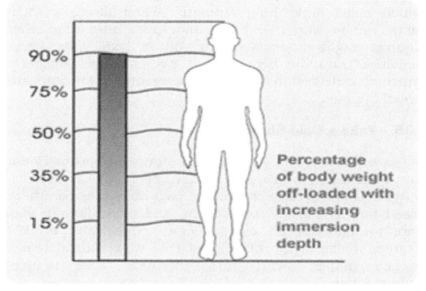

90%
75%
50%
35%
15%

Percentage of body weight off-loaded with increasing immersion depth

The ability to grade the amount of weight off-loaded from joints makes swimming and other water-based activities the ideal option for people who have injuries. Water-based activities are non-weight-bearing, so you can still exercise in the pool when you are non-weight bearing. Just make sure your wounds are healed, and you have clearance from your medical team before going into the water. It can be a safe and comfortable activity for people who otherwise might be very limited in their activities. Exercising in water also increases safety and decreases the risk of losing your balance, falling, and possibly hurting yourself if you were out of the water.

Swimming is probably one of the safest activities for most people. By varying your strokes and body position, you can get a comprehensive full-body workout while swimming. There are many options for workouts to use in the water from aqua jogging, aqua aerobics, swimming, aqua walking, water dumbbell exercises, aquatic games, or just relaxing in the water. Water-based activities are one of the best cardiovascular tasks available as every gallon of water provides 8.25 pounds of pressure on your body when you are submerged in it. The pressure around your body causes you to exert more pressure to be able to breathe, which helps build lung strength. Water-based activities allow you to work the heart and lungs at a time when injuries might otherwise keep you in bed. Water-based activities train the body to use oxygen more efficiently, which is reflected in an improved resting heart rate and breathing rate.

135. Take a Cold Shower

As cold water hits your body, it induces vasoconstriction on your body's surface, and reduces heart rate and cardiac output. This response causes the body to reduce peripheral blood flow, increases metabolism, and blood flow in your core to maintain an average core temperature of 98.6 degrees. Some of the benefits of cold water are increased oxygen intake, heart rate, alertness, and reduced inflammation.

Cold showers can help reduce muscle soreness after a tough workout. Cold showers can also help boost weight loss by triggering brown fat cells to generate heat and start fat burning. Most brown cells are located around the neck and shoulder area, so they are the first to be hit when you take a cold shower.

Coldwater tightens and constricts blood flow, which gives your skin a healthier glow, strengthens your hair cuticles, and doesn't dry out your skin and hair like hot water.

136. Contrast Shower

Hot water activates the parasympathetic nervous system, which relaxes muscles, relieves tension, and soothes muscle fatigue. The hot water also vasodilates the blood vessels in your skin, opens up your pores, releases toxins, and improves skin complexion. The steam from the hot water is also beneficial. As you inhale, the vapor opens airways, loosens up phlegm, clears out your nasal passages, and helps improve symptoms from respiratory illnesses.

However, too much time in a hot shower can damage the keratin cells on the epidermis, the outer layer of our skin. Damaging these cells creates dry skin and prevents the cells from locking in moisture. Lukewarm showers are fine for everyday showering. The best alternative is a contrast shower, where you blend and magnify the health benefits of both the cold and hot shower. First, you get the water as cold as possible and stand in it for one minute. Then, you switch the water to as hot as you can tolerate for one minute. Alternate between one minute each of hot and cold for 3-5 cycles.

The benefits come from the cold water vasoconstricting the blood vessels and circulating all the blood into the middle of your body. Then the hot water is vasodilating (opens) the blood vessels, and all the blood comes rushing out again. The back and forth pumping of the blood through the muscles and organs is excellent for helping with regeneration and detoxification.

K. Shopping for Food

137. Learn to Read Ingredient Lists on Products

People are more health-conscious than ever, so many food manufacturers use deceptive marketing to trick and convince people to eat unhealthy and processed foods which can make it challenging to differentiate between mislabeled junk and healthy foods.

Front labels on products lure people into buying. However, some of these labels are misleading. When you see a product you might want, ignore the health claims on the front of the package. Studies show that these claims fool most people into thinking an unhealthy food is healthy because of the health claims. For example, let's take a look at breakfast cereals which are one of the worst foods for your health. Some will state they are, "Made with whole grains" on the front. Sure, at one point that cereal did start with whole grains, but after processing and adding sugars, it became a Frankenfood and no longer possesses most of the original health benefits. It's almost like saying you could eat a plastic bottle because it's made of plants because millions of years ago there was a forest, which ended up buried, then over millions of years it became petroleum, and that petroleum was processed into a plastic water bottle. It is essential for consumers to read the ingredients list on products they're considering.

Ingredients listed on a label are from highest quantity to lowest. Meaning that the first ingredient has the highest concentration. Pick products that contain whole foods as the first three ingredients as they make up the most substantial part of what you're eating and avoid foods with long lists of ingredients. If you see sugar, refined grains, or hydrogenated oils, in the first three, then it most likely is junk food. Also, if there are two to three lines of ingredients, that too is an indicator that the food is unhealthy.

Be mindful of serving sizes listed on the packaging. Most are misleading and unrealistic. For example, one small bag of chips may say 300 calories per suggested single serving, and the bag is so tiny you assume that the bag is one serving. But when you look at the labeling, you'll be surprised to see that they consider that small bag three servings. So the actual calorie count for the bag is 900 calories. Manufacturers will list smaller serving sizes to mislead you into thinking that the food has fewer calories and less sugar.

Most common healthy product labels:

● Gluten-free (GF): GF foods are processed and loaded with unhealthy fats and sugar. Gluten-free doesn't mean healthy. It says it doesn't contain wheat, barley, spelt, or rye.

● Multigrain: This means that there is more than one grain, not that they're healthy grains. Most of the time, they're unhealthy refined grains unless it says explicitly whole grain.

● Light: These are usually highly processed, watered down, or loaded with sugar to give the food flavor from the fat that was removed.

● Natural: Can be one of the most misleading terms as everything starts as natural. It merely means that one of the ingredients came from a natural origin such as corn, beans, bananas, etc.

● Organic: This doesn't mean that the food is healthier. It means the product is certified to have grown on soil that had no prohibited substances applied to it three years before harvest. These include most synthetic fertilizers and pesticides. Organic produce still has pesticides and synthetic fertilizers, but they're derived from natural sources such as orange peels. According to USDA data, both types of produce are within the level for safe consumption. Research has not demonstrated that pesticides used in organic farming are safer than non-synthetic pesticides used in conventional agriculture. In the end, if the food is processed, it's still most likely unhealthy, and if it's sugar, white flour, or vegetable oils, they still do the same harm to your body.

• Fortified or enriched: Meaning some nutrients have been added to the product. Rice and flours often have B-vitamins added, and milk has vitamin D added. Again, just because something is fortified doesn't mean it's healthy.

• No added sugar: This could be apple juice or orange juice, which are naturally high in sugar and not good for you. It could also mean that unhealthy sugar substitutes were added, which are much worse for your health.

• Low-calorie: These foods mostly have fat removed and replaced with sugar, which is much worse for you. A product labeled low-calorie has to have one-third fewer calories than the original product. These products also require more processing, which lowers the quality of the food.

• Zero trans fat: Actually, it usually means there are less than 0.5 grams per serving. Often the listed serving size is reduced enough to meet the criteria for this label. For example, a large cookie may have 1.5 grams of trans fat, but the company may decide that one serving size is one-third of the cookie and thus be able to say that it is zero trans fat and apply the label even though most people wouldn't eat one-third of a cookie.

• Low-fat: Removing fat from foods and adding sugar in its place to give the food flavor, which is much worse for your health.

• Low-carb: Most foods labeled low carb are highly processed junk foods, similar to processed low-fat foods.

• Made with whole grains: Check the ingredients list and confirm that the whole grains are at least one of the first three ingredients. Otherwise, the product may contain very little whole grains.

• Fruit-flavored: Some processed foods may refer to a

natural flavor, such as cherry soda. However, this doesn't mean the product contains that food, only chemicals designed to taste like it.

Health labels appeal to people's healthy desires. However, these marketing terms mislead people into buying unhealthy products that they think would be good for their health.

138. Avoid Overconsumption of "Healthy Foods"

People assume that foods from "healthy" restaurants and healthier markets are lower in calories, so they tend to eat these types of foods more liberally. Organic foods aren't always healthy or low in calories, even if it's from Whole Foods. If it's in a box, it's still processed, which means it can be readily broken down and absorbed before your stomach can signal to your brain that you're full, which leads to weight gain over time.

139. Avoid Buying Food in Large Volumes

The price of food has decreased and become more readily available, so we eat more of it. Obesity rates have also increased as food prices have dropped. Restaurants and big-box stores have become very efficient at delivering low priced fattening foods.

Stores that sell food in bulk, such as Sam's Club or Costco can help you save money, but they can also help increase obesity. The larger the box, bottle, or bag the food comes in, the larger we think the serving size should be. Studies show that people who buy larger packages of candies, cola, crackers, chips, or just about any food tend to serve themselves more substantial portions. Also, stockpiling bulk foods causes you to eat more in a shorter period. If you're going to buy large containers of food, break up the packages by dividing cookies or chips into smaller bags to help slow down the consumption rate. Also, store the extra portions somewhere out of sight and harder to reach, so you're not looking at them and thinking you need to eat them.

140. Avoid Fat-Free Foods

It seems reasonable to buy fat-free foods if you're trying to lose weight, but they do more harm than good. "Diet" foods are made with artificial sugars like sucralose and aspartame, and other chemicals. Even though diet foods and beverages are lower in calories, sugar-free alternatives have never prevented weight gain. Also, if artificially sweetened foods contain fewer calories than sugary versions, they still trigger sweet receptors in the brain, which causes people to crave and eat more food. Since most people think diet foods are healthier, they think they have room to eat extra servings of other foods, which leads to overconsumption.

141. Shop the Perimeter of the Grocery Store

Shop around the perimeter of stores as an easy way to avoid the expensive and unhealthy convenience foods that are stocked in the front and center. Middle aisles contain packaged and processed foods, which tend to be higher in sodium and higher in calories. That leaves the produce and frozen foods sections, which both offer great low-cost and healthy alternatives.

142. Organic Foods

Organic fruits and vegetables can have one-third of the pesticides of non-organic foods. Organic foods are also less likely to contain residues from more than one pesticide. The real question is, will these small doses add up to an increased health risk down the line over the years and decades. The truth is we're not sure. But we are sure that organic farming is better for the environment, and by supporting it you're forcing chemical companies into creating environmentally friendly alternatives. The pesticides in inorganic fruits and veggies poison the mitochondria in body cells, so it cannot burn fuel, which turns to fat. On average, organic fruits and vegetables may contain 12% more healthy plant compounds than inorganic. Some organic fruits and veggies might contain 20 to 40% antioxidants per calorie than inorganic foods. So, if you are eating five servings of organic produce, it could be like eating six, without consuming any additional calories. Most of the research on whether organic is more nutritious is not conclusive.

On the other hand, organic produce has more natural toxins. Because organic farmers don't use synthetic insecticides and herbicides, organic plants start producing more natural toxins to protect themselves. Unfortunately, these natural pesticides can be just as harmful to people or even worse than the synthetic pesticides used in conventional agriculture. For example, solanine, a substance produced by potatoes as they turn green, can make you ill if you ingest too much of it.

The best option is to thoroughly rinse all fruits and vegetables under running water to remove pesticides and bacteria. Make sure to wash fruits and vegetables with inedible skins, such as citrus fruits and melons, because cutting through the skin will bring contaminants inside.

Toxic chemicals also accumulate in the soil, water, and our bodies. Due to overpopulation, chemicals will continue to be used in agriculture to feed the world population. By purchasing organic, we are contributing less to pollution. If you can afford to pay more and want fewer toxins, buy organic. However, if the higher price is going to prevent you from purchasing produce, buy whatever you can afford. The damage caused by not eating produce is much higher than any you'll experience from eating non-organic foods.

Some people think that eating non-organic food will make them sick due to exposure to pesticides and other chemicals. Fear of pesticides should not keep you from maximizing your intake of produce. For example, some people bypass eating produce that is not organic to eat processed food or meats; that's even worse. You can wash toxins off from produce, but you can't wash it off from meats or processed foods. Meats can have hundreds of times more pesticides, herbicides, and in addition, hormones than produce. So it's just not worth it, eat produce even when it's not organic, and always wash your food so you can reduce chemical levels to trace amounts which may likely never affect your body.

143. Look for Keywords

Whether you're buying groceries or ordering off a menu, look for keywords. Avoid anything labeled fried, creamy, breaded, stuffed, or crispy. Instead, try anything boiled, steamed, poached, and baked. You can significantly reduce the calories in meals by choosing foods that are prepared using healthier cooking methods.

144. Use Self-Checkout

Using self-checkout at grocery stores decreases impulse purchases by 16.7% for men and 32.1% for women when they scan their items and run their credit cards on their own. Typically when you wait in line to pay for your groceries, the lines are lined with unhealthy snacks, which leads to 80% of candy and 61% of salty-snack purchases being unplanned.

145. Don't Shop Hungry

Grocery shopping on an empty stomach can cause you to overbuy food, increase the likelihood of succumbing to cravings for unhealthy food, and inhibits your ability to make smart choices about what you want to eat. Researchers found that fasts can lead people to make unhealthy food choices, picking a higher quantity of high-calorie foods. Eat before going grocery shopping to avoid buying foods that won't help you lose weight.

146. Make a Grocery List

Shoppers who write grocery lists tend to purchase healthier foods and have lower BMI than those who don't. Making a grocery list before going to the market helps keep you organized, which decreases impulse buys of processed foods. Before going to the supermarket, take inventory of what you have in your kitchen and make a list of what you need. Organize it by category so you can get in and get out without having to spend extra time searching, which may lead to purchasing junk food.

147. Avoid Processed Foods

In the US, 57.9% of the food consumed is ultra-processed foods. Ultra-processed foods include bread, soft drinks, packaged snacks, processed meats, take-out food, frozen meals, breakfast cereals, pizza, and foods high in additives and low in unprocessed ingredients. Research shows a correlation between processed foods and developing obesity, cancer, diabetes, autoimmune conditions, and death. An ultra-processed product is made of several processed ingredients like colors, flavors, sweeteners, and emulsifiers. Ultra-processed foods lack nutrients and provide 90% of our added-sugar intake. Substitute a bowl of cereal or Lean Cuisine for a home-cooked dinner, and save your body the damage from eating these foods.

Studies show that people who are on an ultra-processed diet, eat on average 508 calories more each day and gain approximately one pound of body fat per week. People who don't eat ultra-processed foods lose about one pound a week and show an increase in the gut hormone peptide YY, which suppresses hunger and decreases the hunger hormone ghrelin.

Even more interesting is that when the sugars, fat, carbohydrates, protein, and sodium of each diet are compared, they're almost the same. So if someone were to pick up a package of processed food and look at the ingredients, it might not look very bad, and you may buy it, thinking it's ok to eat. The flavors and familiarity of the diets are similar, but people who eat processed food tend to eat faster. They consumed an extra 17 calories, or 7.4 grams of food per minute, more than people eating unprocessed food. Eating faster does not allow your gastrointestinal tract to register the food and signal to your brain that you're full, causing you to overeat. Even though the macronutrient composition of both diets are similar, the unprocessed diet contains more protein and fiber. While the ultra-processed food had more carbohydrates, fat, and was higher in energy density.

148. Eat Nutrient-Dense Foods

Ninety percent of Americans think they eat healthy despite over seventy percent being obese. Disease-causing foods make up most of the standard American diet, with thirty percent of calories from animal products and over fifty percent from processed foods. Processed foods possess only ten percent of the original nutrient content of whole foods. Whole foods are also known as micronutrient foods, such as fruits, veggies, nuts, seeds, and legumes. Macronutrients are everything else.

Micronutrients fuel the immune system's proper functioning and enable the detoxification and cellular repair mechanisms that protect us from chronic diseases. The nutrient density of your diet will determine the nutrient density in your body's tissues. Studies show that focusing on food quality, such as eating nutrient-dense foods rather than calorie counting, is the easiest way to lose weight.

Dr. Mark Fuhrman developed this nutrient density scale to help people select a nutrient-dense diet and lose weight faster.

1000	KALE	119	GRAPES	34	SALMON
1000	COLLARD GREENS	119	POMEGRANATES	31	EGGS
1000	MUSTARD GREENS	118	CANTALOUPE	31	MILK, 1%
1000	WATERCRESS	109	ONIONS	30	WALNUTS
1000	SWISS CHARD	103	FLAX SEEDS	30	BANANAS
895	BOK CHOY	98	ORANGE	30	WHOLE WHEAT BREAD
707	SPINACH	98	EDAMAME	28	ALMONDS
604	ARUGULA	87	CUCUMBER	28	AVOCADO
510	ROMAINE	82	TOFU	28	BROWN RICE
490	BRUSSELS SPROUTS	74	SESAME SEEDS	28	WHITE POTATO
458	CARROTS	72	LENTILS	28	LOW FAT PLAIN YOGURT
434	CABBAGE	65	PEACHES	27	CASHEWS
340	BROCCOLI	64	SUNFLOWER SEEDS	24	CHICKEN BREAST
315	CAULIFLOWER	64	KIDNEY BEANS	21	GROUND BEEF, 85% LEAN
265	BELL PEPPERS	63	GREEN PEAS	20	FETA CHEESE
205	ASPARAGUS	55	CHERRIES	12	FRENCH FRIES
238	MUSHROOMS	54	PINEAPPLE	11	WHITE PASTA
186	TOMATO	53	APPLE	11	CHEDDAR CHEESE
182	STRAWBERRIES	53	MANGO	11	APPLE JUICE
181	SWEET POTATO	51	PEANUT BUTTER	10	OLIVE OIL
164	ZUCCHINI	45	CORN	9	WHITE BREAD
145	ARTICHOKE	37	PISTACHIO NUTS	9	VANILLA ICE CREAM
132	BLUEBERRIES	36	OATMEAL	7	CORN CHIPS
127	ICEBERG LETTUCE	36	SHRIMP	1	COLA

149. Avoid Canned Food

If you have the option, fresh or frozen foods are always preferred over canned foods. Overall, canned foods can provide nutrient levels similar to those of their fresh or frozen counterparts. It's essential to read the label and ingredient list because canned foods can be high in salt, sugar, or preservatives that are sometimes added to canned foods to improve their flavor, texture, and appearance.

The cans used for canned foods are often lined with plastic that may contain BPA, a chemical associated with weight gain, heart disease, and type 2 diabetes.

150. Hang a Mirror by Your Dinner Table

Scientists have found that eating unhealthy food in a

room with a mirror was less appealing than in a room without one. Also, when given a choice between a healthy and unhealthy dish, most people opted for a healthy meal, which means that the presence of a mirror makes unhealthy foods less appealing. Hang one in your kitchen to discourage the consumption of sweets and other unhealthy foods.

Having to watch yourself eat something harmful makes you responsible for your choice and triggers discomfort brought on by deeply ingrained social standards. This phenomenon only applies if you opted to eat unhealthy food, not with healthy eating.

151. Clean Your Palate

People crave seconds for sweets or other high-calorie foods when the taste lingers in their mouths. To cleanse your palate, eat a mint or gum to remove the flavor from your mouth. Not only will this get rid of the taste from your mouth, but it will also keep your mouth busy. Drinking tea, water, or another beverage also helps remove the flavor from your mouth.

152. Plate Your Food to Help You Lose Weight

Most meals consist of animal protein as the main dish with small sides of veggies and starches. Instead, rearrange your plate, so vegetables are the main dish with smaller sides of meat and carbohydrates. By rearranging your plate, you'll automatically eat fewer calories and consume more healthy vitamins and nutrients.

153. Eat off a Red Plate

We eat less when there is a higher contrast in colors between the plate and your food. Color and contrast can cue your appetite, determine how much you eat, and ultimately how much weight you gain. If you eat off a plate with more contrast, such as a red plate, you'll eat less. In comparison, diners will serve themselves more food if the color of their food matches the color of their plate. So, if you're eating from a white plate, you're more likely to serve yourself more rice or pasta. Research has shown that people who eat off red dishes eat much less, possibly due to the association with the color red with stop signals and other human-made warnings. Therefore the color red may trigger a stop reaction, and you end up eating less food.

154. Eat off a Smaller Plate

People tend to eat all of the food they place on their plate. You could lower your caloric intake with minimal effort by reducing the size of your plate, which would cause you to load less food onto your plate. By allowing your plate to control your portion size, you can lose over 10 pounds a year or more (the average dinner is 800 calories).

Another way to look at it is instead of using the average size plate of 11-12 inches, use a 9-10-inch plate, which would reduce the amount of food you serve yourself by 23%. Using a smaller spoon to eat with or a smaller serving spoon can cut 14% off of each meal, leading to additional weight loss. Using smaller plates tricks your eyes and brain into thinking you're eating more so you get full faster.

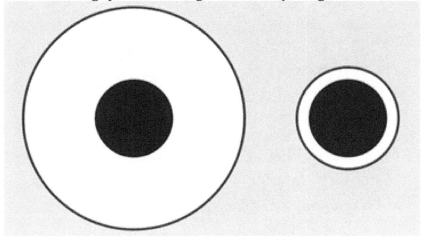

155. Use Smaller Plates and Larger Cups

When you are hungry, you want to fill your belly. Using larger cups for teas, water, or other calorie-free beverages during meals will encourage you to drink more liquids overeating solid foods that are usually higher in calories. Filling your stomach with more liquids will reduce appetite, calorie intake, prevent overeating, and help you lose weight.

156. Use a Portion Control Plate

Portion control plates are a simple way to give yourself a visual guide serving yourself a nutritious plate. The plate outlines the correct portions of protein, fruit, vegetables, grains, and even dessert. Portion plates give you visual size indicators for adjusting portions and eating essential food groups without the guesswork.

You can construct your portion control plate with a permanent marker by making one quarter of your plate fruits, veggies, grains, and proteins.

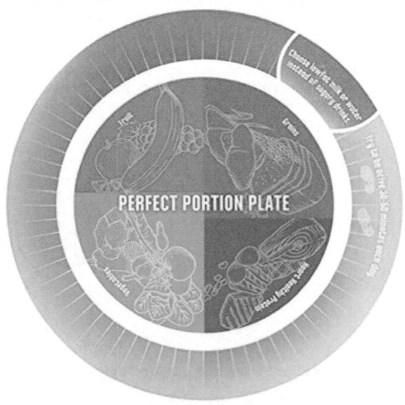

157. Avoid Crash Diets

Crash diets will give you short term results, but not long term. Don't sabotage your long term weight loss goals by going on a crash diet. Crash diets rob you of the ability to make real habit changes. Generally, to lose weight you don't have to eat less. You have to eat healthily.

To lose one pound per week, you'll have to lose 3500 calories a week or 500 calories a day. Count calories and trim portions, but don't eat less than 1,200 calories a day or you'll actually slow your metabolism by 20% per day, and your body will start burning muscle for energy. The less muscle you have, the fewer calories you'll burn overall.

L. Everyday Foods for Weight Loss

158. Eggs

The American Dietary Guidelines Advisory Committee no longer recommends that we limit dietary cholesterol. Research has shown that it has little effect on blood cholesterol levels. Make omelets with the entire egg. The yolk contains metabolism-boosting nutrients, fat-soluble vitamins, essential fatty acids, and choline, a powerful compound that prevents your body from storing body fat around your liver. Eating eggs for breakfast can increase your feeling of fullness and cause you to eat fewer calories for up to 36 hours automatically. Eggs are inexpensive, readily available, and can be prepared in a matter of minutes. One issue to be aware of is that chickens are raised in cramped conditions, so they have to be fed antibiotics daily to keep them from getting sick and hormones to grow faster. All of these chemicals get translated into the eggs, which are absorbed by your body when you consume them.

159. Eat Beans

Beans and legumes are high in protein and fiber, contributing to feelings of fullness and lower calorie intake. Eating one serving a day of peas, beans, lentils, or chickpeas helps manage blood sugar levels. They also contain resistant starch which stays in your intestines longer keeping you satiated.

Some people have difficulties tolerating legumes and get gas after eating them. To help avoid this issue, soak beans in water overnight, which activates enzymes that digest the sugars in beans that cause gas and increases the protein content. You can also add herbs such as epazote or baking soda to beans to break down some of the beans' natural gas-making sugars. Another strategy is to rinse canned or soaked beans, discard the soaking water, and use fresh water for cooking the beans, effectively draining out the amount of gas-producing sugars.

160. Eat Dark Chocolate

Dark chocolate contains healthy fats, antioxidants, prevents cavities, and slows the absorption of sugar into the bloodstream. This helps prevent an insulin spike after a meal, which would otherwise push sugar straight into your fat cells. Insulin spikes prevent fat-burning and make you hungry several hours later, which can cause insulin resistance and diabetes.

This only works if you eat chocolate with at least 70% cacao. White and milk chocolate is loaded with sugar and is bad for you. Eat one square of dark chocolate the size of your thumbnail 20 minutes before and five minutes after a meal to cut your appetite by up to 50%. Eating a piece of dark chocolate before a meal triggers hormone that tell your brain that you're full, so you eat less.

161. Oatmeal

Oatmeal is a weight loss superfood, high in protein, low in calories, lowers cholesterol, and high in fiber, so it passes slowly through your digestive tract. Oatmeal itself can help you lose weight because it will help you feel full longer than other foods, and the high fiber increases the number of calories you burn each day. Steel-cut oats are the type of oatmeal with the most elevated protein and fiber content. Although the nutritional difference between quick oats, old fashioned oats, and steel cuts oats is negligible. Soaking raw oats in water or any milk overnight (overnight oats) are easier to digest than cooked oats.

162. Spirulina

Spirulina is a single-cell, microscopic blue-green algae that is one of the earliest forms of life on the planet. Spirulina is a high-protein seaweed supplement that's typically dried and sold in powdered form. Dried spirulina is 60% protein and a complete protein. One tablespoon has 4 grams of protein and a day's requirement of vitamin B12, which can encourage weight loss by giving you more energy, boosting your metabolism, boosting your immune system, and increasing weight loss. Spirulina is considered a "superfood" due to its vast array of nutrients, including protein, essential fatty acids, vitamins B, C, E, and chlorophyll.

Often, when you feel hungry, your body is creating the effect because it is looking to fill its own need for nutrients. When you feed yourself poor-quality foods regularly, your brain will trigger your appetite to find what it wants. Spirulina will increase the concentration of nutrients in your body and can reduce hunger and cravings in the process. The protein in spirulina has a high bioavailability, which allows it to be absorbed four times greater than beef which makes spirulina ideal for building muscle which in turn helps you burn more calories.

Spirulina is a rich source of Omega-3 fatty acids and gamma-linolenic acid (GLA). GLA can help regulate blood sugar and control insulin levels, which will minimize carbohydrate binging and help you lose weight. Spirulina helps with high cholesterol, high triglycerides, attention deficit hyperactivity disorder, fatigue, viral infections, and cancer.

M. Vegetables

163. Eat more Vegetables

If your body requires 2100 calories a day, you'd have to eat 420 celery stalks, 105 carrots, and 26 eggs or only 1¼ cup of peanut butter to meet your daily energy needs. Therefore filling up on veggies causes you to consume much fewer calories and lose weight. Wherever possible substitute veggies for meats in dishes. For example, swap squash for beef in lasagna.

Increased consumption of high-fiber vegetables increases weight-loss, compared with diets low in high-fiber foods. Not only are these veggies super-satiating, but they're also full of anti-inflammatory antioxidants and will displace high-calorie snacks like nutrient-deficient potato chips and pretzels.

164. Purslane

Purslane is a weed that grows in many parts of the world and can be eaten raw or cooked as a highly nutritious vegetable. Purslane is much higher in omega-3 fatty acids than other greens. In addition, it contains high amounts of ALA and trace amounts of EPA, a more biologically active form of omega-3. Purslane is loaded with vital minerals, including potassium, magnesium, and calcium. Research shows that purslane's high fiber and high nutrient density help promote weight loss.

165. Cilantro

Cilantro is a superfood high in protein, calcium, magnesium, manganese, potassium, vitamins A, C, E, and K, and B vitamins. It is a natural diuretic that detoxifies the kidneys, liver, and tissues. It reduces bloat and water retention, promotes weight loss, and stabilizes blood sugar. These attributes all help you feel satiated, help with digestion, and helps restore natural gut flora. Cilantro leaf takes more energy to digest then it does to eat it, so it's a negative calorie food.

Cilantro leaf contains oil that helps get rid of the intestinal fungus, yeast, and bacterial infections that limit weight loss. The leaf lowers blood pressure and high cholesterol levels, improving your circulatory system and metabolism. It also contains polyphenols that eliminate fat cells from the liver, which helps people get rid of fat deposits faster as they diet.

The high iron content in cilantro leaf helps purify the blood and improve kidney and liver function, promoting weight loss

Cilantro is high in zeaxanthin, lutein, and cryptoxanthin, which help prevent blindness and keep small arterioles healthy which prevent cellulite, diabetic neuropathy, and bloating. It also has quercetin, which lowers cholesterol and high blood pressure, and improves metabolic function

The cilantro leaf is high in fiber and chlorophyll, which helps detoxify body cells, prevents the kind of inflammation that discourages exercise, and causes weight gain.

166. Eat Chili Peppers

Adding chili peppers to meals can help you lose weight by raising your metabolism and burning away fat. Capsaicin is the active ingredient in peppers that makes them hot. The heat generated by peppers can increase your consumption of stored calories and oxidize layers of fat.

Eating ground red pepper or chili peppers causes thermogenesis, which speeds up your metabolism. Thermogenesis is the heat created by your body as it digests foods and accounts for 10-15% of all of the calories you burn in a day. Only eating 0.9 grams (1/10 of a teaspoon or a small pinch) of ground red pepper with a meal will cause you to eat 16% fewer calories because the heat created by the chili increases satiety.

As we age, we lose our taste buds, eating peppers intensifies flavors, making eating more pleasurable while helping you spike your metabolism, lose weight, and increase your sense of fullness. Fullness is one of the primary reasons that capsaicin works.

167. Rhubarb

Rhubarb is a vegetable that is high in fiber, vitamin C, vitamin K, potassium, manganese, calcium, polyphenols (which can act as antioxidants), zeaxanthin, and lutein. Rhubarb is low in calories, high in fiber, aids in weight loss, improves circulation, prevents Alzheimer's, fights cancer, improves digestion, helps manage diabetes, and helps lower cholesterol. Rhubarb increases the effect of iron from dairy products, which causes the body to store less fat and has a laxative effect, which aids in weight loss. Additionally, the fiber helps you feel full faster, which can further reduce total caloric intake and promote weight loss.

168. Eat Zoodles

Zucchini noodles look like spaghetti but are a nutrient-dense, low-calorie, and natural alternative to traditional wheat noodles. Eating zoodles over pasta cuts out 480 calories for every two cups of pasta, while two cups of zucchini noodles have 66 calories and twice the fiber. Zoodles taste just as good as a bowl of spaghetti, and they can quickly help you achieve your weight loss goals. Zucchini noodles can be made in minutes using a zucchini squash and a five-dollar spiralizer.

169. Spaghetti Squash

When you're in the mood for pasta or lasagna dishes, spaghetti squash is a healthy replacement. It has 75% fewer calories than a cup of plain pasta and has a much lower glycemic index. Spaghetti squash is low in calories, high in fiber, very nutritious, and helps promote weight loss.

170. Bell Peppers

Peppers are low in calories, starch, and loaded with vitamins A and C, potassium, folic acid, fiber, and the spicy ones have capsaicin. Bell peppers start green, turn yellow, orange, and then red. The fully ripened red ones have almost 11 times more beta-carotene and 1.5 times more vitamin C than the green ones. Vitamin C counteracts stress hormones, which trigger fat storage around the midsection. They also reduce cholesterol and lower blood sugar to help control appetite.

171. Beets

Beets are a nutrient-dense superfood that can help boost longevity, aid in weight loss, prevent Alzheimer's disease, and prevent chronic diseases, like cancer. Beets are high in fiber, vitamin C, magnesium, folate, and can add years to your lifespan if consumed regularly.

Beetroots lower cholesterol, are high in fiber which helps improve digestion, and can help you lose weight. Beets increase levels of testosterone, a hormone that promotes fat tissue loss and increases muscle mass, and are rich in magnesium which improves nerve and muscle functioning. As your muscle mass grows, the extra muscle burns more calories than fat, helping you lose weight. Beets contain phytonutrients known as betalains (betanin and vulgaxanthin), which are useful in reducing inflammation, detoxing, and supplying the body with antioxidants.

Beetroot is loaded with nitrates, which are converted into nitric oxide by the body. Nitric oxide vasodilates blood vessels, which increases blood flow, resulting in 16% more stamina during physical activity. Because it lowers cholesterol, increases erections for men during sexual intercourse, and helps them last longer in bed, it has earned the title of "Nature's Viagra." The phytonutrients in beets, like betalains, are cancer-preventive.

Beets are also considered brain food that slows the effects of dementia and Alzheimer's disease. The high-nitrate content of beets increases blood flow to the white matter of the frontal lobes of the brain, regions linked to degeneration from dementia and other cognitive disorders. Folic acid also protects against Alzheimer's by preventing damage to the hippocampus, which the brain devotes to memory and learning.

172. Broccoli

One cup of broccoli contains 30 calories, which means you would have to eat 11 cups of broccoli to equal the calories in one cup of pasta. One cup of raw broccoli gives you 100 percent of your daily vitamin C and vitamin K, contains folate, vitamin A, vitamin B6, and potassium.

Broccoli has several nutrients that help with weight loss. Vitamin C is used to synthesize the amino acid carnitine, which is essential for metabolizing fats into energy. People who don't consume enough vitamin C will burn less fat during exercise.

Calcium stimulates the breakdown of stored fat, reduces the production of new fat cells, and prevents some fats from being absorbed by binding with them in the intestine. Consuming calcium and vitamin C together will boost your metabolism.

Chromium helps regulate the activity of insulin. Through this function, it helps carbohydrate metabolism and increases weight loss. One cup of cooked broccoli has 22 micrograms of chromium, which is about two-thirds of the recommended daily intake.

One cup of broccoli has five grams of a special type of fiber that increases the digestion, absorption, and storage of food. Finally, broccoli has sulfur-containing phytochemicals named sulforaphane and indole-3-carbinol that trigger fat burning weight loss.

N. Fruits

173. Apples

Eating one medium-sized apple with its skin on contains over 4 grams of fiber, which is about one-fifth of our daily need. Apples are high in pectin, a potent fiber that slows the digestion of food and makes you feel fuller with fewer calories. Studies show that eating apples or pears before meals will help you eat fewer total calories, resulting in significant weight loss.

174. Stone Fruits

Stone fruits, also known as drupes, are seasonal fruits with a fleshy exterior and a pit or stone inside. They include cherries, nectarines, plums, and peaches, which fight inflammation and protect against diabetes, metabolic syndrome, heart disease, and obesity. The stone fruits' natural compounds work on different cells in the body, including fat cells, immune cells, and cells that line the circulatory system, to protect them from aging and disease. Stone fruits have a low glycemic index, low-calorie, and high in nutrients like vitamins C and A, which help people lose weight. It's best to eat ripened stone fruit. As they ripen, the nutrient content increases.

175. Tart Cherries

Sweet and tart cherries both contain naturally occurring anthocyanins and other flavonoids, but tart cherries have more per serving. Therefore tart cherry juice is much healthier. University of Michigan researchers completed a 12-week study with rats that were fed tart cherries and found that they lost 9% of their belly fat over those fed a western diet. The researchers believe this is caused by tart cherries' high anthocyanin content, a flavonoid with potent antioxidant and anti-inflammatory activity.

176. Passion Fruit

Passion fruit is almost one-third fiber and has enzymes,

which help lower cholesterol, regulate your blood sugar, keep your gut healthy, and detox your body. The seeds inside contain piceatannol, a chemical that improves blood pressure and insulin sensitivity. The fruit is high in vitamins A, C, E, iron, and potassium.

The high Vitamin A and beta-carotene content in passion fruit help fight inflammation, improve eyesight, and boost your immune system. Vitamin C will help protect the pituitary gland from damage and helps your skin retain its elasticity after losing weight. Vitamin E reduces joint pain so that you can exercise without pain, and it also improves your body's general metabolic function. The combination of antioxidants in passion fruit help dissolve fat deposits and reduce cellulite.

Iron helps keep your body well oxygenated so you can function at peak performance. It is also necessary for cellular respiration and detoxification. Potassium helps regulate your blood pressure and metabolism. Passion fruit is also high in magnesium, copper, and phosphorus, which are vital to your neurological system, prevents dry skin, and hair loss that often happens during dieting.

177. Banana

Bananas are very versatile, convenient, and are an excellent substitute for energy bars, which often contain lots of sugar and chemicals. Some types of bananas can be added either raw or cooked to a wide variety of dishes. Although bananas are more calorie-dense than most other fruits, they are also more nutrient-dense, supplying potassium, magnesium, manganese, fiber, numerous antioxidants, and vitamins A, B6, and C.

Some people avoid bananas when trying to lose weight due to their high sugar and calorie content. Even though a banana contains 27 grams of carbs on average, it can still help prevent weight gain because it's low in calories (105) and has three grams of fiber. Bananas have a low glycemic index, fight muscle cramps, reduce swelling, regulate weight, control insulin levels, keep blood pressure low, help overcome depression, and prevent acidity.

Studies show that eating one banana per day reduces your blood sugar, especially for diabetics and cholesterol levels.

The levels of nutrients increase in bananas as they ripen. Bananas with dark spots are eight times more effective in enhancing your immune system than green-skin bananas. Also, the riper the banana gets, the thinner and sweeter the peel becomes. That's because of ethylene, a natural plant hormone that fruits release as they ripen. Ethylene interacts with the sugars and fiber in the banana skin, changing complex sugars into simple sugars and breaking down pectin, a fiber in bananas that keeps them stiff. That's why the older your banana is, the flimsier it feels. At the same time, other hormones break down the green pigments in the peel, turning them yellow and eventually brown.

In most western countries, we are used to tossing banana peels in the trash, but in most other countries, people take advantage of their nutritional benefits. It is high in vitamin B6 and B12, magnesium, potassium, and some fiber and protein. Banana peels also have several bioactive compounds like polyphenols and carotenoids.

Before eating a banana peel, wash it to remove pesticides. Banana peels are typically cooked, boiled, fried, eaten raw, or put in a blender for shakes. They are not as sweet as the banana flesh but become sweeter as the peel ripens. When added to a shake, the skin is almost unnoticeable, and it gives your shakes a delicious thick texture like an ice cream shake.

178. Kiwifruit

One kiwi has as much vitamin C as three oranges. It also has vitamin E, folate, prebiotic fiber, and a natural enzyme called actinidin that aids in digestion by breaking down protein in the body. Studies note that kiwi can help control blood sugar, improve cholesterol, feed good gut bacteria, and increase weight loss. Studies also show that eating two kiwis a day will decrease your waist size 1 cm per month.

179. Grapefruit

Grapefruit was made by crossing a pomelo with an orange in the 18th century, and is high in pectin. Half a grapefruit has only 39 calories but provides 65% of the recommended daily intake (RDI) of vitamin C, and red grapefruit has 28% of the RDI vitamin A. It also has folic acid, potassium, and lycopene, a phytochemical that protects arterial walls from oxidative damage.

Grapefruit has a very low glycemic index (GI), which means it releases sugar into your bloodstream slowly helping you lose weight, reduce body fat, and decrease the consumption of food. Studies show eating half a grapefruit about 30 minutes before meals reduces calorie intake, lowers cholesterol, lowers blood pressure, and decreases body weight by 7.1%.

180. Guava

Guavas are one of the highest protein fruits available. They also are high in vitamin C, lycopene, manganese, folate, potassium, fiber, and are high in water content. The combination of high protein and fiber helps slow digestion, which helps keep you satiated longer, preventing you from overeating, regulating your metabolism, and gaining weight. Guavas are low in sugar compared to other popular fruits such as oranges, grapes, and apples. They also have about 12% of your dietary fiber needs, which improves digestion and further promotes healthy weight loss.

181. Pomegranate

Pomegranate is high in vitamins like B, C, K, and fiber. It also has punicalagin, a chemoprotective compound that reduces carcinogens from binding to cells. Its antioxidants help guard against heart disease, lower cholesterol, and improve immune function. Pomegranates contain nitrates that are converted to nitrite, which causes vasodilation, and, subsequently, more blood flow throughout the body. This increased blood flow improves memory, athletic performance, and recovery after exercise. Pomegranate also has polyphenols and conjugated linolenic acid, which helps burn fat, boost your metabolism, and suppress appetite.

182. Watermelon

Watermelon is 90% water, which helps the body stay hydrated, helps you feel full, reduces cravings between meals, and makes you lose weight. A 100-gram serving of watermelon has only 30 calories. It's also high in arginine, an amino acid, which burns fat, and decreases fat accumulation.

Watermelon rinds and seeds also have significant health benefits. They're high in fiber, vitamins B and C, and high in citrulline, a compound linked to multiple health benefits. In particular, citrulline converts to arginine, which is vital to the heart and improves circulation by dilating blood vessels which improves oxygen delivery to muscles and improves exercise performance.

183. Berries

Berries are very high in antioxidants, fiber, nutrients, and water, yet they are low in "energy density," or concentrated calories, to help you feel full and satisfied after eating. Berries are also high in polyphenols, a powerful chemical that decreases the formation of fat cells and eliminates abdominal fat. Some berries such as boysenberries, black raspberries, marionberries, red raspberries, and strawberries are super-antioxidant foods with high oxygen radical absorbance capacity (ORAC) values. Berries are high in vitamin C. Dark-colored berries are high in ellagic acid, which kills some types of cancer cells. Raspberries are a rich source of ketones which increase antioxidants that burn fat cells.

Berries get their bright color from anthocyanins, a type

of flavonoid from the polyphenol class of phytonutrients. Anthocyanins are potent antioxidants known as radical scavengers. They help fight oxidation, a natural process associated with heart disease, cancer, and aging.

184. Avocados

Avocados are a type of berry from Mexico, but unlike strawberries or other berries, they have only one seed. Avocados are high in vitamins C, E, K, potassium, and folate. They also contain niacin, riboflavin, copper, magnesium, manganese, antioxidants, and contain almost 20 times more fat-soluble phytosterols than other fruits. Avocados are also the fruit with the highest fat content 15% by weight. They contain high amounts of heart-healthy monounsaturated fats similar to those found in olive oil.

Avocados are a superfood, especially for weight loss. Because avocados are high in fiber and fat, they help you feel satisfied and keep you feeling full longer. The fats are burned at a higher rate than other types of fats, increase fat burning, cause calorie burning after eating, and reduce appetite and decrease the desire to eat after a meal. Studies show a 40% decrease in appetite for several hours and decreased belly fat storage after eating half an avocado.

185. Tomato

Tomatoes are a fruit that is rich in vitamins A, B6, and C, fiber, protein, iron, lycopene, manganese, and potassium. They help reduce water retention and fight leptin resistance. Being leptin resistant will make it difficult to lose weight. Tomatoes are low in calories around 22 calories for an average size tomato and an appetite-suppressant. Because they are a "high-volume" food, they have large amounts of air, water, and fiber. Tomatoes are a filling low-calorie substitute for high-calorie dairy and meats. Eating tomatoes will make you feel full, cut down your calorie intake, and create a calorie deficit required to lose weight.

Ernesto Martinez

O. Grains

186. Gluten-Free Products

Gluten is a generic name for the proteins found in wheat (wheat berries, spelt, durum, semolina, emmer, farina, graham, farro, einkorn, and Khorasan wheat), barley, rye, and triticale (a cross between rye and wheat). Gluten gives food structure; it acts as a glue to help foods maintain their shape.

Up to 6% of the world population has gluten intolerance. People with celiac disease can't tolerate gluten, and even a small crouton is enough to cause trouble. Gluten causes the immune system to attack and damage the small intestine, prevents the absorption of nutrients from food, causes nerve damage, osteoporosis, seizures, and infertility. Some people are gluten sensitive, which causes similar symptoms and weight gain. In these cases, cutting out gluten from your diet would be beneficial and can lead to weight loss due to the reduction in inflammation and water retention.

Gluten-free products are beneficial for those who need them, but they're not any healthier than foods that contain gluten. Gluten-free foods tend to be highly processed, more expensive and will yield little to no benefit to most people who do not have a gluten intolerance. Gluten-free diets aren't all automatically better for you. Gluten-free (GF) labeled foods tend to have more calories, extra fat, and added sugar for flavor.

187. Kamut Wheat

Khorasan wheat is an ancient grain, also known as Kamut. It's full of omega-3 fatty acids, protein, and is low in calories, but not gluten-free. Kamut has 30% more protein than regular wheat, reduces cholesterol, blood sugar, and cytokines, which cause inflammation. If you're going to eat wheat, eat Kamut, it is rich in protein, fiber, zinc, magnesium, and offers a variety of potential benefits.

188. Make White Rice Healthier

Reduce the calories in a bowl of white rice by 60%. Add one teaspoon of coconut oil to every half cup of white rice. After it's cooked, store in the refrigerator for 12 hours, and serve either cold or reheated. As the rice is cooled, the sugars in the rice start forming tight bonds called "resistant starch." As mentioned previously, this starch is resistant to digestion, so the body is not able to absorb many calories. As the rice cooks, the fat from the oil seeps into the rice and makes the rice even more resistant to digestion.

189. Swap Out your Rice

My good friend Spencer once told me he had to eat white rice every day, or he felt weak. White rice is a staple food for many people, but it has low nutritional value, is high in toxic arsenic (all types of rice, especially brown rice), and it has a high glycemic index, so it promotes weight gain.

Fortunately, there are several alternatives such as:

- **Riced Cauliflower**

Ricing the fiber-filled, low carb, and low-calorie veggie is an alternative to rice. Cauliflower is high in vitamin C, potassium, and even plant-based protein. Plus, riced cauliflower's texture is so similar to rice that you'll barely notice the difference.

- **Chopped Cabbage**

Chopped cabbage is low in calories and carbs with a mild flavor that combines with many styles of cuisine. It's an excellent source of vitamins C (31% daily value) and K (68% daily value), in a 1/2-cup (75-gram) serving. Vitamin K is essential in blood clotting and bone health.

- **Quinoa**

Quinoa is a seed, is gluten-free, and much higher in protein than rice. A 1/2 cup (92-gram) serving of cooked quinoa has double the protein (4 grams) of rice. Quinoa is a complete protein, so it has all nine essential amino acids that your body needs. It's also high in magnesium and copper, which are crucial to energy metabolism and bone health.

- **Freekeh**

Freekeh is made from unripened green wheat grains. A 1/4 cup (40-gram) serving has 8 grams of protein, 4 grams of fiber, and 8% of the daily value for iron, which is needed to create healthy red blood cells

- **Shirataki Rice**

Shirataki rice is made from konjac root, which is native to Asia and rich in a unique fiber called glucomannan. A 3-ounce (85-gram) serving of shirataki rice is calorie-free and has glucomannan, which forms into gelatin in your stomach and helps keep you full for long periods.

- **Farro**

Farro is similar to barley but has larger grains and is a whole-grain wheat product. It's used similarly to rice, but it has a nuttier flavor, chewy texture, and more protein.

- **Whole-Wheat Couscous**

Couscous is a type of pasta used in Mediterranean and Middle Eastern cuisine. Whole-wheat couscous is rich in fiber and protein. Couscous pearls are smaller than grains of rice, so they add a unique texture to foods.

- **Bulgur Wheat**

Bulgur wheat is made of cracked pieces of whole-wheat grains. It's similar to couscous, but it is not pasta and is a good substitute for rice. Bulgur wheat is 76 calories in 1/2 cup (91 grams), about 25% fewer calories than an equal serving of white rice.

- **Barley**

Barley is similar to wheat and rye, but looks identical to oats and has a chewy texture and earthy taste. A 1/2 cup (81-gram) serving has about 100 calories, about the same as an equal serving of white rice, yet it is higher in protein and fiber. Also, barley has a variety of nutrients, 10% of the DV for niacin, zinc, and selenium.

- **Buckwheat**

Like quinoa, buckwheat contains all essential amino acids and is a good substitute for oats, rice, and flour if ground into a fine powder. Buckwheat is not wheat; it's a flower, and the edible portion is a seed produced. It's high in fiber, protein, and contains a lot of bioavailable antioxidants, and is rich in many trace minerals, including manganese, magnesium, and copper.

- **Riced Broccoli**

Similar to riced cauliflower, broccoli is low-carb and low-calorie. A 1/2 cup (57 grams) serving has only 15 calories, 2 grams of fiber, and vitamin C (25% DV).

P. Nuts and Seeds

190. Pistachios

Pistachios are low in calories, healthy fats, fiber, protein, antioxidants, and various nutrients, including vitamin B6 and thiamine. Their health effects include weight loss, monounsaturated fatty acids that help control cholesterol and blood sugar, and improved gut, eye, and blood vessel health. De-shelling pistachios helps prevent you from popping one too many nuts and overloading on calories.

191. Flaxseed

Flax, also known as linseed, can be ground into flaxseed meal or used as an oil. Flaxseed is rich in fiber, which helps clean your intestines and improve digestion, stabilize blood sugar, and promote weight loss.

Flax seeds are high in omega-3 fatty acids, which reduce inflammation, lower cholesterol, fight autoimmune diseases, reduce the risk of cancers, and improve cardiovascular support.

Flaxseed also has a particular type of fiber called lignans that reduce blood pressure, aid in weight loss, and supports kidney health.

When consuming flaxseeds, don't eat raw or unripe flax seeds as they contain compounds that can cause indigestion. Also, make sure to grind up your flax seeds because your body has difficulty digesting the skin of the flaxseed, and most of the nutrients are inside the seed. If you're using flax seeds in any form, make sure you stay hydrated because the excess fiber can result in stomach cramps and constipation.

192. Almonds

Eating almonds helps you burn fat and lose weight. Almonds are high in protein, healthy monounsaturated fats, omega-3 fatty acids, and fiber. Almonds are rich in L-arginine which can help you burn more fat and carbs during workouts. Eat a handful of almonds before heading to the gym.

Q. Top Items to Avoid for Weight Loss

193. Avoid Fluoride

Fluoride is a mineral found naturally in bones, water, soil, plants, and rocks. Fluoride is used in dentistry to strengthen teeth and help prevent cavities.

During World War II, public health experts were looking for inexpensive ways to keep the general population well and to have healthy citizens that could work in factories and fight the war. One of those strategies was fluoridation, adding fluoride to drinking water and dental products. Fluoride in low concentrations decreases the frequency of dental caries cost-effectively. The ADA (American Dental Association) says that every $1 invested in water fluoridation saves $38 in dental treatment costs.

Even though fluoride is a naturally occurring compound, it can still cause side effects when consumed in large doses. Some of the dangers include fluorosis (leaching of minerals from bones), low IQ scores in children, bone cancer, arthritis, kidney disease, damage to the brain's frontal lobe, and thyroid gland. The thyroid gland is found in the neck, regulates the metabolism, and many other body systems. An underactive thyroid can lead to depression, weight gain, fatigue, and aching muscles. Children tend to be more affected by fluoride because they're more likely to swallow toothpaste, which contains significantly more fluoride than fluoridated water. Over 95% of western European countries have removed fluoride from their drinking water due to health concerns, yet most large cities in the USA still fluoridate their drinking water. You can reduce your exposure by filtering your drinking water and using fluoride free dental products.

194. Household Chemicals

After losing weight, some people start regaining much of what they lost. Research has shown that some of this weight gain may be due to chemicals in clothing and furniture. Synthetic chemicals called perfluoroalkyl and polyfluoroalkyl or PFASs found in consumer products make it difficult for people to lose weight by slowing the metabolism.

These chemicals are found in nonstick cookware, water-repellent fabrics, grease-proof food packaging, cleaning supplies, and personal care products. Almost half of grease-proof paper wrappers and 20% of cardboard containers, like pizza boxes, contain PFASs that can leach into food. PFASs accumulate and stay in the body for a long time, causing multiple medical problems, including low infant birth weight, thyroid disease, and reproductive issues. PFASs are also known to interfere with hormone systems in the body.

Avoid cleaning products that contain carcinogens, reproductive system toxins, neurotoxins, and allergens. Use natural, non-toxic cleaning products to avoid all of these. Also, avoid breathing volatile organic compounds (VOC), which are the vapors that come from paints, lacquers, thinners, glues, cleaning supplies, nail polish, markers, fuel, office equipment, inks, and pesticides. VOC's accumulate in closed spaces and can be up to ten times higher indoors than outdoors. VOC's can have short and long term health effects.

Dr. Bronner's has a variety of safe and healthy products that can be used to clean your home and self-care.

195. Avoid Car Odors

Since the industrial revolution, we have introduced over 80,000 chemicals to create many of the things surrounding us in our daily lives. Unfortunately, exposure to many of these chemicals can alter our body chemistry, interfere with our metabolism and cause weight gain even when eating a healthy diet.

The "new car smell" is an example of a scent that many of us recognize and even look forward to smelling. However, that "scent" you are breathing in daily is most likely formaldehyde and benzene, which can cause adverse health effects, weight gain, and even cancer. These persistent organic pollutants (POPs) are toxic chemicals that adversely affect human health and the world's environment. POPs can increase the risk of weight gain and even type 2 diabetes independent of calorie intake.

The materials used to build cars, from hard and soft plastics to adhesives, textiles, and foam, create the smell of a new car. These materials contain chemicals that slowly seep into the air (known as 'off-gas') you breathe. The heat from a vehicle left in the sun can speed up the release of these toxic chemicals, and it slowly decreases over time as the car gets older.

These volatile compounds will build up in small spaces, such as inside a car; when someone gets into a car and closes the door, especially after being in the hot sun, they're inhaling the build-up of toxic chemicals into their body. The longer your commute, the more you are likely to be exposed to these cancer-causing carcinogens that risk reproductive and developmental health. The amount of carcinogens in your car depends on temperature, ventilation rate and type, humidity, solar radiation, cabin value, vehicle age and grade, car upholstery material, and travel distance.

When you park your car, always leave the windows slightly cracked so air can ventilate in and out. When you get into your vehicle, roll down your windows and drive for a few minutes to air out the cabin before closing the windows and turning on the air conditioning. During your commute, keep your windows open as much as possible. Unless you're in traffic, close your windows and recirculate the air in your car to prevent breathing car exhaust, which is worse. Every once in a while, open the windows to dilute these chemicals' concentration inside your vehicle.

Limit your exposure to toxic chemicals because your bodies cannot keep up with the constant daily barrage of environmental and dietary toxins.

WARNING

MOTOR VEHICLES CONTAIN CHEMICALS KNOWN TO THE STATE OF CALIFORNIA TO CAUSE CANCER AND BIRTH DEFECTS OR OTHER REPRODUCTIVE HARM. These chemicals are contained in many vehicle components and replacement parts, vehicle fluids, and paints and materials used to maintain vehicles, including, but not limited to, fuel, oil, batteries, brakes, and wheel balancing weights. In addition, motor vehicles emit engine exhaust and fumes, and when serviced, cleaned or maintained generate used oil, waste fluids, fumes, grease, grime and particulates from component wear, which contain chemicals known to the State of California to cause cancer and birth defects or other reproductive harm.
(Posted in accordance with Proposition 65 in Calif. Health & Safety Code §25249.5 et seq.) For further information about Proposition 65: www.oehna.org/prop65.html.

196. Avoid Plastics

Numerous studies are demonstrating that exposure to chemicals used in plastics, preservatives, pesticides, and flame retardants, are causing metabolic disorders, including diabetes and obesity.

Obesogens are artificial chemicals that disrupt normal endocrine function and cause obesity. The most commonly affected hormone is estrogen. Exposure to chemicals found in plastics hampers fat mobilization during fasting, making it harder to lose weight when on a low-fat diet.

- **Bisphenol-A (BPA)**

Bisphenol-A (BPA) is widely used in many types of plastics, baby bottles, plastic food and beverage containers, and metal food cans. BPA's resemble estradiol, a form of the female sex hormone estrogen. As a consequence, BPA binds to estrogen receptors inside the body, causing 96% of pregnant women in the US to test positive for BPA.

BPA exposure has been linked to insulin resistance, heart disease, diabetes, neurological disorders, cancer, thyroid dysfunction, weight gain, obesity, and genital malformations.

- **Phthalates**

Phthalates are used to make plastics flexible and soft. They are found in food containers, toys, plastic bottles, beauty products, flooring, pharmaceuticals, shower curtains, and paint. Phthalates leach out of plastics and contaminate foods, the water supply, and even the air we breathe. Most Americans test positive for phthalate metabolites in their urine. Phthalate exposure is linked to endocrine disruption, weight gain, diabetes, and genital malformations in boys.

- **Dibutyltin (DBT)**

Dibutyltin (DBT) salts are used to make PVC (vinyl) plastics used in construction materials (window frames and vinyl flooring), and medical devices (tubing and packaging). DBT is found in seafood and house dust, indicating that DBT exposure is widespread. DBT is linked to obesity and diabetes in people.

- **Perfluorooctanoic Acid (PFOA)**

Perfluorooctanoic acid (PFOA) is used in non-stick cookware made with Teflon and microwave popcorn. PFOA has been found in the blood of over 98% of Americans. It is linked with thyroid disorders, obesity, low birth weight, and chronic kidney disease.

How to Reduce Your Exposure to Obesogens in Plastics.

Avoid food and beverages stored in plastic containers. Use stainless steel, glass, or quality aluminum water bottles instead of plastic. Use glass bottles for babies. Instead of non-stick cookware, use cast iron or stainless steel. Use natural cosmetics. Use glass, wood, or ceramic when possible, and don't use plastic wraps.

If you use plastic, do not heat up, microwave, store acidic foods like tomato sauce, place them in direct sunlight, or wash them with harsh soaps. All of which can facilitate the leaching of chemicals from the plastic into your foods.

197. Wash Your Hands Instead of Using Hand Sanitizer

Hands down washing your hands for at least 20 seconds by rubbing your hands together to create friction, is the most effective way to kill a broad spectrum of germs. However, when soap and water are not available, use alcohol-based hand sanitizer, sanitizer is an effective alternative.

Many hand sanitizers, unfortunately, contain a germ-killing chemical called triclosan, which is an "obesogen," a substance that causes weight gain by disrupting your body's hormones. Researchers found that people who had detectable levels of triclosan in their bodies were associated with a 0.9-point increase in their BMIs. Research has shown that triclosan can damage the endocrine system, reduce muscle strength, and weaken the immune system.

198. Use the Right Cookware

The federal drug administration has shown that a group of over 5,000 toxic chemicals known as per- and polyfluoroalkyl substances (PFASs) are in our food and water supply. Ninety-eight percent of Americans have PFAs in their blood, and research shows our diets are the primary source of these compounds. PFAs are in plastic cooking utensils, nonstick cookware, food packaging, cleaning products, and other industrial products that have leached into our food and water supply. They are also contaminating our livestock and sewage sludge used for fertilization. These "forever chemicals" are linked to liver damage, certain types of cancers, thyroid disease, infertility, high cholesterol, obesity, and several other health conditions.

In particular, nonstick cookware and plastic cooking utensils leach PFAs at a faster rate and in a more substantial amount into your food when heated. Research shows that avoiding or reducing PFAs exposure can help people (especially women) maintain stable body weight after weight loss. PFAs are known as "obesogens" because they can upset body weight regulation. People with higher levels of the chemical in their blood have slower metabolisms. Research has shown that after being on a diet for six months, women with the highest amounts of PFAs in their blood gained between 4 lbs. and 5 lbs. more than everyone else.

199. Best Cookware to Use

- ### Cast Iron

Cast iron cookware has been relied upon for cooking since ancient times. It's heavy but versatile, durable, inexpensive, and the safest cookware available. Some iron does leach into food when cooking and especially when acidic foods, like tomato sauce, are prepared. Cast-iron pots and pans shouldn't be put in the dishwasher or washed with detergents, and they rust if left wet. To maintain a cast-iron pan, rinse with warm water and a brillo pad. You also have to season the pan by rubbing oil on the cooking surface and heating the pan up for 5-10 minutes to allow the oil to seep into the metal. Once the pan is seasoned, it will have excellent non-stick properties.

- ### Glass

Glass is an inert material, so nothing reacts with it or leaches from it. Pyrex is the gold standard for cookware. But you have to follow instructions for using glass cookware, or it could shatter.

- **Stainless Steel**

Stainless-steel cookware is durable, doesn't react with food, easy to clean, and can be washed in the dishwasher. More expensive stainless-steel pots and pans have an inner core of aluminum or copper that helps food cook more uniformly. Expensive cookware has a nonstick option, while inexpensive versions require oil, so food doesn't stick.

- **Copper**

Good quality heavy-gauge copper pots and pans can last a lifetime. They're prized for their ability to cook foods evenly, however, copper can also leach into food, especially acidic foods, causing a metallic taste. Trace amounts of copper can be beneficial for you and isn't generally a health problem. Copper toxicity is rare in healthy individuals, but it can occur in people with Wilson's disease, a rare genetic disorder. Copper cookware lined with stainless steel is an option that eliminates the leaching problem.

R. Junk Food

200. Potato Chips and French Fries

Potato chips are the number one food contributing to weight gain. While eating a serving of french fries is worse for your body than rum and six times worse than cigarettes. French fries and potato chips are both linked to significant weight gain. These foods are typically high in salt, which causes you to continue eating them even after you're full.

Fried, baked, or roasted potatoes also contain cancer-causing substances called acrylamides. Consider whole boiled potatoes as a healthy alternative to help fill you up.

201. Substitute Salads for Potatoes

If you want to stick with your weekly burger, substitute the fries for a salad. Doing so will prevent you from eating more at your next meal, save over 150 calories, and fill you up faster with fiber-rich veggies that are good for digestion.

202. Switch From White Potatoes to Sweet Potatoes

Both types of potatoes are healthy if prepared healthily. Sweet potatoes, however, have more fiber and are lower on the glycemic index than white potatoes. Sweet potatoes have around 4 grams of protein, 25% of the day's fiber, and 11 times the recommended daily allowance of vitamin A.

203. Swap Veggies for Corn Chips

There's nothing like the crunchy texture of corn tortilla chips. Unfortunately, they're deep-fried and high in calories. A healthy option is to cut corn tortillas into quarters and bake them in the oven. They will have the same crunchy texture that most people enjoy. Another option is to cut up crunchy baby carrots, celery sticks, or cucumber slices to dip into sauces, hummus, or salsa. Veggies are high in fiber, nutrients, and low in calories.

204. Pastries

Pastries, cookies, and cakes are typically made with artificial trans fats to help prolong shelf life, refined flour, and sugar. All of these ingredients cause weight gain, are linked to multiple health problems, are high in calories, and are not very filling. Eating these low-nutrient, high calorie foods will cause you to become hungry very quickly. Avoid foods high in sugars and refined sugars which cause your blood sugar to crash. Instead, eat complex carbohydrates such as whole grains, protein, and a little fat with each meal to keep your blood sugar steady and help you stay full longer.

When you're craving something sweet, reach for a piece of fruit, some protein, or a piece of dark chocolate instead.

205. White Bread

White bread is highly refined, contains added sugar, and has a high glycemic index. Eating white bread can cause you to overeat as it spikes your blood sugar levels. Eating two slices of white bread per day will increase your risk of obesity by 40%. Remember, the whiter the bread, the faster you'll be dead. If you like bread, try Ezekiel bread, which is probably the healthiest bread on the market.

206. Avoid Wraps

Flour tortillas and flat pita bread, also known as wraps, may seem like a healthier, lower carb alternative to a sandwich, but they're not. Some are comparable to bread, and many are higher in calories because they need more fat to hold the flour together and make them pliable. They can have as many carbs and calories as four or five slices of bread. Instead, try an open-faced sandwich, to help reduce caloric intake.

207. Corn Versus Flour Tortillas

When you go out for Mexican food, corn tortillas (50 calories) are always going to be a healthy alternative to flour (140 calories). Corn tortillas have more fiber, whole grains, and other nutrients while being lower in fat and calories than flour tortillas. Over centuries Mesoamericans genetically modified corn (or maize) from its origins as an inch-long bundle of dry seeds into the cobs of succulent kernels we know today.

One plain ear of corn has approximately 100 calories, similar to an apple. And with nearly 3 grams of fiber per serving, corn helps you feel full longer, so you're less likely to overeat and put on the pounds.

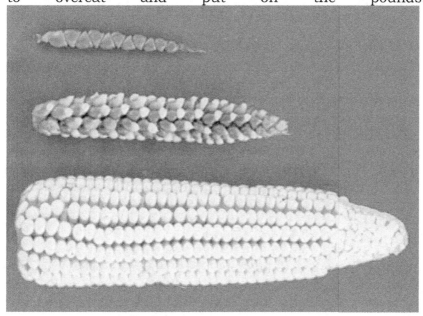

Without corn, it would be impossible to feed the over 7.8 billion people we have on our planet. Corn is one of the oldest examples of genetically modified organisms (GMO) which have become controversial. Humans have been genetically modifying foods and animals to help perpetuate preferred traits. For instance, Chihuahuas and Great Danes are genetically modified wolves. Humans genetically modify themselves with vaccines and gene therapy to treat illnesses that could wipe out the human race. Plants are modified to help them resist diseases, grow larger and faster, and make them drought tolerant. Without GMO plants and the foods that come from them, we would not be able to feed the world population we now have. The Earth can only support one billion people, but with technology, petroleum, and GMO foods, we've been able to surpass that number. GMO crops can yield multiple times more food in less time and with less land than non-GMO foods. Due to overpopulation, the less GMO food we eat, the more rainforest we have to cut down.

Over 99% of the food you eat in restaurants and fast food has some GMO ingredients in it. Processed foods are also high in GMO foods, so these days it's almost impossible to avoid GMO foods even if you wanted to.

In 2015 a Pew Research Center survey showed that 90% of scientists from the American Association for the Advancement of Science believed that GMOs are safe to eat. But more than 50% of U.S. adults think they're not safe. People debate which foods should be labeled GMO, whether they should be labeled, and the long-term effects of producing and eating them will have on our planet and our bodies. There is little evidence that eating GMO food is bad for you, but there is ample evidence that it is necessary due to overpopulation.

208. Avoid the Bread Basket

Substitute bread baskets for a bowl of nuts or a side salad to cut down on calories. Warm dinner rolls with butter are delicious, but they're loaded with calories and bad carbs. Another strategy is to eat healthy snacks before leaving home to keep you satiated so you're less likely to crave unhealthy foods.

209. Candy Bars

Candy bars are high in calories, low in nutrients, and not very filling. An average-sized candy bar has 200–300 calories. Candy bars are made of unhealthy ingredients such as vegetable oils, sugar, and refined flour. Candy bars are even strategically placed in stores so consumers are tempted into impulsively buying them. If you are looking for a snack, eat a handful of nuts or a piece of fruit instead.

210. Breakfast Cereals

Breakfast cereal is loaded with sugar, making them one of the worst breakfast habits. Even though they say "whole-grain" or "low-fat," the first ingredients are usually refined sugar and grains. Cereals can be tricky, when you examine the ingredients, they can seem healthy, but after processing, they can often be as bad as eating a candy bar.

211. Pizza

Pizza is one of the most popular and unhealthy foods consumed. They're high in calories and often contain unhealthy ingredients like highly refined flour and processed meat. For example, one slice of Costco pizza has 750 calories. As an alternative order pizza from places that make healthier pizza or make your own pizza. Making your pizza allows you to pick healthier ingredients and avoid processed ingredients high in preservatives and sugar.

212. Go Thin, Not Deep

Deep-dish or pan-style pizzas are much higher in calories and fat than regular pizzas. A thin-crust slice can have over 350 fewer calories than a regular hand-tossed slice. Most pizzas are made with refined white flours, loaded with calories, and known to boost your cravings throughout the day due to high amounts of salt.

S. Meats

213. Eat Less Animal Protein

People are taught that eating animal protein is healthy, but we don't worry about protein when eating junk food. But as soon as someone starts eating healthy, they worry about getting enough protein. Saturated fat, salt, and sugar are the nutrients that cause the most damage to your body, and are found in the highest concentrations in animal products and processed foods.

You'll often hear people say they only eat white meats because they're healthier than red meats. That is a myth; all meats do not have fiber, are high in protein, and are high in environmental pollutants. One type of meat is not healthier than the other, except that larger animals have higher concentrations of contaminants. They are larger, so they have to eat more and therefore are exposed to higher doses of environmental pollutants.

People who eat a high-protein vegetarian meal, typically eat 12% fewer calories in their next meal than people who eat meat. Start with substituting one animal protein-based meal a week for a plant-based meal. Also, plant-based diets tend to have more fruits, vegetables, grains, beans, legumes, and nuts. These are richer in fiber, vitamins, and other nutrients. Vegetarians generally eat fewer calories, have less fat, weigh less, and have less chronic diseases than nonvegetarians.

If you do prefer to eat meat, free-range and grass-fed are healthier alternatives, but they're the most ecologically unsustainable and do the most damage to the environment. The cows, chickens, and pigs will be happier, but the fact is the planet is overpopulated, and 70% of arable land in the world is already used to grow food for livestock. Rainforests are being cut down to have the massive amounts of additional property needed to feed grass-fed and house free-range animals. Because we have 7.8 billion people to feed, the food choices we make will determine our fate. Ninety one percent of land burned in the Amazon is by livestock producers.

When Patrik Baboumian, one of the strongest men in the world was asked, "How are you as strong as an ox if you don't eat meat?" He answered, "Have you ever seen an ox eat meat?" People who eat a plant-based diet can build muscle and strength just as effectively as people who eat animal protein.

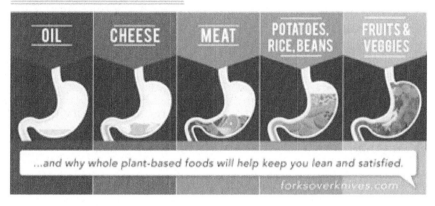

CALORIE DENSITY WHAT 500 CALORIES LOOK LIKE

OIL | CHEESE | MEAT | POTATOES, RICE, BEANS | FRUITS & VEGGIES

...and why whole plant-based foods will help keep you lean and satisfied.

forksoverknives.com

214. Processed Meats

Eating processed meats and unprocessed red meat causes weight gain of about a pound per year and increases your risk of death from all causes by around 3%. Highly processed foods do not satisfy hunger as well as less processed, higher fiber foods, creating a higher total intake of calories. Also, processed meats like bacon, sausage, hot dogs, and bologna usually contain nitrate, nitrite, and N-nitroso compounds, potent carcinogens that can induce tumors. Additionally, they typically contain high amounts of salt, which can irritate the stomach lining and increase the compounds' carcinogenic effects.

215. Boil Meats

Cooking meat helps break down tough fibers and connective tissue, making it easier to enjoy, chew, and digest. It also leads to better nutrient absorption, and it kills harmful bacteria such as Salmonella and E Coli. The best way to cook meat (chicken, fish, pork, and beef) and even eggs is by boiling. Boiling meats helps preserve higher concentrations of protein, which is often denatured, and also becomes more toxic when using other cooking methods. The fats contained in the flesh are easily dissolved and leached out into the boiling water, thus making the food leaner, healthier, and easier to digest.

216. Beef

If you must eat beef as a source of protein, grass-fed beef is healthier, but it is also less sustainable and causes more damage to the environment. Choose leaner cuts of prime rib, ground beef, or T-bone steak, which are amongst the healthiest cuts because they contain more heart-healthy omega-3 fatty acids than most fish. Keep red meat consumption to no more than two three-ounce servings per week to keep your gut healthy and pick low-calorie seasonings.

217. Marinate Meats in Beer

Marinating meats for four hours in black beer (dark lager) before cooking will reduce carcinogenic compounds in the flesh. Other types of beer and wine are also helpful, but not as effective as dark beer. Cooking meat at high temperatures produces carcinogenic compounds in the meat called polycyclic aromatic hydrocarbons (PAHs). PAHs are extremely toxic to humans and increase the risk of multiple forms of cancer. Due to the antioxidants in alcohol, soaking the meat for four hours in black beer marinade before cooking resulted in reducing the formation of PAHs by 68%, pilsner by 36.5%, and nonalcoholic beer by 25%.

218. Fish

Fish are a lean, high quality source of protein. Fish have multiple health benefits and provide one of the best sources of fatty acids known as omega-3s. These fatty acids help prevent waist-widening inflammation and heart disease. Protein enables you to maintain muscle mass, therefore reducing excess fat accumulation. Some of the best seafood include salmon, mussels, bluefish, and Atlantic mackerel. Buy wild-caught fish over farm-raised seafood when possible and check out the National Resource Defense Council (NRDC) website to make sure you're eating sustainable seafood. Due to overfishing, over 90% of large fish in the oceans have perished. Five to twenty times more sea animals are killed as by-kill in the process of catching fish such as tuna. By-catch and by-kill are unintended animals caught by accident in fishing gear, and can include marine mammals, sea birds, sea turtles, and sharks.

Farm-raised fish are more sustainable but have as much as 20% less protein compared to wild fish. They're also higher in polychlorinated biphenyl (PCBs), a cancer-causing chemical often found in farm-raised salmon at a concentration 16 times higher than is found in wild salmon, and dioxin, a highly toxic carcinogen at 11 times higher than usual amounts.

T. Technology

219. Use your iPhone to Keep Track of your Meals

Some people eat well 90% of the time, but it's the 10% that derails them. People often exaggerate the healthy foods they eat and underestimate the bad stuff. For example, you eat well all day and then grab handfuls of high-calorie samples at Costco. To keep a more accurate journal of what you eat, take a picture of everything you eat each day and log into your food log later. Hopefully, this will help you not forget those extra snacks in the lunchroom at work or a friend's house.

220. Air Fryer

If you love fried foods, air fryers are a healthy alternative. Air fryers have a fan that pushes heated air (up to 400 F) around the food, similar to a convection oven. The circulating air makes the outside of the food crispy and keeps the inside soft, like deep-fried foods. A container below the frying basket catches any grease that drops. Air frying cuts fat and calories by 70% to 80% compared to frying in oil and helps reduce the amount of the chemical acrylamide in fried potatoes by 90%.

Cutting out fried foods will also cut your risk of heart disease, type 2 diabetes, and cancer.

An air fryer can cook almost anything that you would typically fry in oil, such as:

- Vegetables
- Chicken, including chicken fingers and nuggets
- Onion rings and french fries
- Fish
- Doughnuts

Some models also have a toasting feature and bake like a conventional oven, which allows you to bake brownies or roast a chicken.

221. Keep a Food Journal

Multiple studies show that people who keep food journals are more likely to succeed at losing weight and keeping it off. Some studies have demonstrated that people who keep daily food journals lose twice as much weight as people who keep weekly records. Writing down and reviewing what you ate for the day every day helps you be conscientious of how much you're eating. Although it's very simple to do, this is one of the activities that most people resist. On average, you'll spend less than 12 minutes a day. There are also multiple smartphone apps and websites to help you keep your journal.

222. Use Chopsticks

Eating with chopsticks will slow down your eating. When you eat slower and take small bites of food, your gut will have time to signal to your brain when it's full, helping you avoid overeating. Your stomach gets full before your brain has time to release the signal to stop eating. Chopsticks will help you avoid this as you'll be forced to eat at a slower pace allowing you to stop before you go from starving to stuffing yourself.

223. Purchase a Fruit Bowl

Keep a fruit bowl in plain sight on your desk or in the middle of your dinner table, so you're more likely to grab fruits and veggies over unhealthy options. Pears, Bananas, apples, plums, and oranges keep well without being refrigerated. Reaching your goal of eating the recommended five to nine daily servings of fruits and veggies can make it easier to lose weight. Having a visual reminder like a fruit bowl helps make it happen.

224. Start Using a Scale Daily

Once you start using a scale daily, you'll have improved awareness of your weight, be more conscious of what you eat, and adjust your behavior daily when you see the pounds creeping up. Many people are in fat denial; they avoid scales, buy stretchy or loose clothes that hide their weight, or hide in the back of pictures. Using a scale can help encourage weight loss by providing a level of accountability. The best time to weigh yourself is every morning after going to the restroom and before eating breakfast. Weigh yourself naked or with bedtime clothing, but be consistent. Weighing yourself also helps develop your mindfulness skills and body awareness. People who weigh themselves daily on average will lose 17 lbs. a year, regardless of whether they try any other strategies.

225. Use a Pedometer

Most people walk much less than they think they do. Using a pedometer on your iPhone, such as the free health application, allows you to keep track of your steps. This simple technique has helped my patients make remarkable gains in weight loss and increase their activity level. When you first start using your pedometer, you'll notice that your readings may only be 4000 or 5000 steps per day. If you sit at work or you are sedentary at home, the number could be lower. Checking into your pedometer during the day will help you stay motivated to increase your daily step total. Pedometers are a simple way to increase your activity for better health, improved fitness, and weight loss.

Studies show that people who walk less than 5,000 steps a day are more likely to be overweight, while people who walk more than 9,000 daily are prone to be of healthy weight.

Every 2,000 steps are approximately equal to one mile.

> o   1,000 steps = a half mile
> o   4,000 steps = 2 miles
> o   10,000 steps = 5 miles

226. Light Therapy Lamp

If you're unable to get outside during the day due to your work schedule or a disability, try using a UV free light. It mimics the full spectrum of light found in daylight and can deliver the recommended amount of daily sunlight requirements without the risk of sunburn as it is UV-free. Studies show that fat cells are sensitive to sunlight. Therefore, sitting in the sun can result in decreased lipid droplet size and increased fat breakdown (basal lipolytic rate). The sun's blue-light spectrum, a spectrum that can penetrate the skin, can cause fat cells that lie just beneath our skin to shrink. Researchers have shown that daily exposure to sunlight can help one to stay slim or become slim. In contrast, reduced sunshine can lead to weight gain.

227. Toilet Bench

Toilet stools can promote a more natural position for moving the bowels. Studies show that a squat-like position with the knees positioned above the hips is better for naturally moving the bowels. Sitting on a modern toilet can cause a kinking-effect in the colon when seated with knees positioned at a 90-degree angle to the torso. Sitting on a toilet and placing your feet on a toilet bench puts you into a squatting position, fully extending the colon and helping the bowels void.

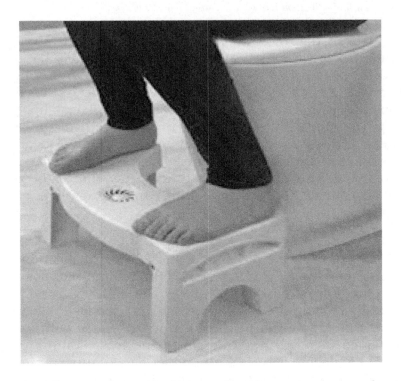

A toilet stool can help people who experience chronic constipation, hemorrhoids, and inflammatory bowel disease, and can also help anyone who wants to maintain healthy bowels and reduce the chances of experiencing these problems.

Patients with chronic constipation may feature microflora changes of the large bowel, characterized by a relative decrease in obligate bacteria and a parallel increase in potentially pathogenic microorganisms and fungi. This condition causes chronic low-grade inflammation.

Studies show that inflammation causes weight gain, difficulty losing weight and is a common underlying factor in all major degenerative diseases, including cancer, heart disease, hypertension, and diabetes.

A month-long study involving 52 people — 41.1 percent of women who had a mean age of 29 years — shows a toilet stool helped a majority of them:

- Seventy-one percent reported faster bowel movements.
- Ninety percent reported less straining.
- After the study, two-thirds said they would continue using toilet stools.

U. Eating Out

228. Eat at Home

Eating out is a convenient and time-efficient way to fuel up for a busy day in our fast-paced modern culture. However, restaurant food is generally served in large portions, packed with calories and fat, and is usually made of the lowest quality ingredients to increase profit margins.

People who eat at restaurants consume 200 calories per day more than those who prepared all their meals at home, and those who ate in sit-down restaurants consumed more calories than people who ordered from fast-food restaurants. People who dine out, also consume more sugar, saturated fat, and sodium, so preparing and eating at home is much healthier.

Full-service and fast-food restaurants — the two largest segments of the commercial foodservice market — account for about 73.1% of all food-away-from-home sales in 2019. Full-service establishments have wait staff, and, perhaps, other amenities such as ceramic dishware, non-disposable utensils, and alcohol service. In contrast, fast food restaurants use convenience as a selling point; they have no wait staff, menus tend to be limited, and dining amenities are relatively sparse. According to the National Restaurant Association, restaurants are the Nation's second-largest private-sector employer, providing jobs for one in 10 Americans.

229. How to Eat Out

Eating out with friends and family is a necessary social experience. However, if you're going to eat out, you must develop skills needed to eat out without consuming excess calories and gaining weight from restaurant food.

How to reduce your calorie intake when eating at out:

- Ask your server not to bring bread or chips to the table. Order a low-calorie appetizer or drink a low-calorie beverage such as water instead.

- Split meals with others and an extra dinner salad.
- Eat healthier throughout the day in preparation for a night out at a restaurant.
- Eat a healthy snack before you go into the restaurant.
- Read the menu carefully and be selective about what you order. Perhaps an appetizer and a dinner salad are all you need.
- Cut portions of high-calorie condiments like sauces, salad dressing, or gravy by asking them to be placed on the side.
- Only spend calories on foods you like. If you don't like pasta, then substitute it for veggies.
- Eat mindfully appreciating the sight, texture, and taste of your food while slowing your consumption rate.

People who use these strategies during mealtime can reduce their daily calorie intake by about 297 calories a day, of which 124 of those calories are from restaurants.

230. Go Protein Style

When you order a hamburger, ask for a lettuce bun or protein style, which means hamburger meat, cheese, tomato, onion, pickles, ½ sauce, and wrapped in lettuce. Protein style can help you cut down on carbohydrates and save around 150 calories by switching from a bread bun to lettuce. Most restaurants offer this option.

231. Appetizers

Adding a healthy appetizer such as an apple, salad, or a bowl of broth-based soup before eating out can reduce your dinner's total calorie intake by 20%. Use your appetizer to fill up, so you don't eat as much during meals.

232. Pack a Lunch

Packing a lunch instead of eating out is an excellent way to save money and eat healthier. But it also makes it easier to manage what you eat and control your portion sizes.

Preparing your lunch gives you calorie-cutting power, rather than in the hands of the restauranteurs who have no stake in your weight-loss. A meal at a standard sit-down restaurant can average more than 1,100 calories.

233. Order off the Kids Menu

If you're craving a hamburger and fries or want portion control in a fast-food restaurant, try ordering from the children's menu. Serving sizes have grown so much that today's children's portions are the same size as past adult portions. Try ordering a McDonald's Happy Meal to satisfy cravings without hurting your weight loss goals.

234. Avoid Combo Meals

Fast food restaurants often offer "combo" or "value meals" that are usually less expensive and made to make you think you're getting a better deal. However, these meals are even worse for your health. "Value" or "combo meals," bundle soft drinks, french fries, cookies, or other high-calorie sides that add hundreds of calories to your meal. By ordering items bundled together, you're likely to buy more food than you need or want, and end up overeating as a result. To help prevent overeating, only order the items you want to eat one by one.

235. Avoid Value Menu Items

"Value menu" items are reduced price food items on a fast-food restaurant menu, meant to attract new customers and get them to spend at different price points. A successful "Value Menu" item, such as a Mexican pizza or hamburger, has to satisfy several factors to be a success. It has to have a low price, taste good, and be big enough to make the customer feel they're getting a good deal. Restaurant chains such as McDonald's, Taco Bell, or White Castle have mastered the Value Menu and built their empires on their success.

Unfortunately for customers, "Value Menu" items are high in sodium, fat, cholesterol, calories, low in fiber, and have very little costly fruits and vegetables. "Value menu" items average 1,000 mg of sodium, 400 calories, and 21 grams of fat. Another danger with "Value menu" items is that their low price encourages you to buy several high-calorie items at once.

236. Avoid Fast-Food

The US Department of Agriculture says that approximately 37% of US consumers' money goes to eating outside the home. McDonald's alone feeds 25 million Americans a day at its more than 14,000 US locations or close to 8% of the population.

Fast food restaurants strongly incentivize those large amounts to entice consumers. A person can pick between an 8 oz drink or a 40 oz drink, but often more substantial portions are the best bargain. A hungry person will often not make the best nutritional choices and will succumb to marketing campaigns.

However, "fast food" is not just the food in fast-food restaurants. Fast foods include cookies, chips, breakfast cereals, soda, candy bars, french fries, burgers, white flour baked goods, pizza, and other high-calorie, processed low-nutrient foods. Fast foods have identifiable characteristics: they're quickly and easily accessed, come out of a bag, can, or box, and are ready to eat without having to be prepared. Fast foods are made to be eaten and absorbed quickly into the bloodstream. These foods have multiple chemicals, synthetic ingredients, are calorically dense, highly flavored, and nutritionally barren. Fast foods are made of low-quality ingredients such as MSG, corn syrup, artificial sweeteners, sugar, coloring agents, salt, and other potentially disease-promoting chemicals.

Flooding your bloodstream rapidly with calories can have significant biological effects. For example, if you ate a 200 calorie muffin, the muffin would be metabolized into simple sugars (glucose), which would enter the bloodstream in 5 to 10 minutes, rapidly increasing insulin levels remaining in your blood for hours. On the other hand, if you ate 200 calories of beans, the carbohydrates from the beans would take longer to digest, and these calories would slowly enter the bloodstream over hours. Therefore, eating beans would release small amounts of glucose into the blood each minute, which would require only a minimal amount of insulin to deal with this amount of sugar. Exposing yourself to excess sugar and white flour products accelerates aging and chronic disease. In 2019, the share of food at home was 45.2%, and food away from home was 54.8%.

Shares of total food expenditures

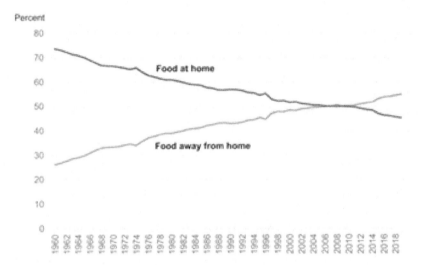

Source: USDA, Economic Research Service using data from the Food Expenditure Series (FES), nominal expenditures.

V. Eating at Home

237. Change Up Your Salads

Eating the same salads every day can be boring. Vary your ingredients by using different veggies, cheeses, nuts, proteins, and dressings. Salads are a valuable tool in helping you reach your weight loss goals. Salads are excellent as an appetizer to help you eat less during meals and increase satiety.

238. Boredom Eating

Boredom can be bad for your brain by decreasing memory and mental acuity. However, it also causes you to gain weight, stripping you of your ability to make smart food choices and making you into an emotional eater. Emotionally eating can cause you to overeat or prioritize less nutritious foods over those your body needs. Eating out of boredom almost always happens when we're not in the physiological need for food. After the first couple of bites, whatever you're eating won't even feel satisfying because you weren't starving in the first place. To prevent boredom eating, engage in physical or mental activity to keep you busy.

239. Dress Up Your Meal

I can remember having breakfast with a friend and ordering pancakes. It was an unhealthy option to start with, and was only the beginning of my eating misadventure. The restaurant only offered margarine and pancake syrup made of high fructose corn syrup to sweeten the hotcakes.

If you're going out to eat at a place where you know they don't offer healthy options, consider bringing your own to improve your meal's nutritional content. For example, bring grass-fed butter to a restaurant that you know serves margarine; extra virgin olive oil, or balsamic vinaigrette for your salad dressing if it only offers unhealthy soybean oil-based options; an avocado, or healthy herb seasonings as a salt alternative. Thinking ahead can help you avoid having to eat high calorie or unhealthy condiments to enjoy your meal.

240. Increase Fiber Intake

Fiber helps you lose belly fat and reduce appetite by slowing the movement of food through the gut. Fiber, unlike other foods, is not digested in the small intestine. Instead, it is moved into the large intestine, where fermentation occurs. This difference increases fullness for more extended periods, slows digestion, increases nutrient absorption, and prevents constipation. Simple ways to add more fiber to a balanced diet is increasing consumption of fruit, legumes, whole grains (oats and brown rice), and eating vegetables.

One type of fiber, viscous fiber, is only found in plant foods such as beans, oat cereals, brussels sprouts, flax seeds, asparagus, oranges, and the weight loss supplement glucomannan. When viscous fiber mixes with water, it forms a gel. This gel stays in your stomach longer, increases nutrient absorption time, and reduces appetite and food intake.

241. Try Meal Prep

Depending on your eating habits, meal prepping can help some people lose several pounds a week. Having a food routine can help keep you from impulse eating. Meal-prepping can help you save on groceries, save time, eat healthier, and reach your weight-loss goals. Making meals in batches for the week helps you plan, save time, and stay on your healthy eating plan. Having homemade meals and snacks readily available can help you avoid drive-thrus and convenient, processed foods.

242. Make Your Food Picture Perfect

The current trend of taking pictures of your food and posting them on Instagram or Facebook has led to people making better food choices. This has three benefits. The first is the fear of social shaming. Not many people want to show themselves eating unhealthy food, especially when they have weight or health problems. Second, making your food look picture-perfect can encourage you to pick healthier, more colorful vegetable choices. Thirdly, people who spent time preparing the food they eat, tend to enjoy their food more than food that is prepared for them, even if the food was considered "healthy."

243. Chew Food Thoroughly

Chewing food thoroughly slows down the rate that you're ingesting food, reducing calorie intake, and causing weight loss. After each bite of food count the number of times you chew, this is a good way to start chewing your food longer. Chewing is also vital to digestion, and by slowing the intake of food, your stomach will have more time to increase gut hormones that signal to your brain that you're full and helps reduce calorie intake.

244. Brush Your Teeth

After eating a meal, if you feel an urge to continue eating, put your napkin over your plate, push it away, get up, and brush your teeth. Brushing your teeth will help cut down on in-between snacking, decreasing your appetite, and helping you avoid overeating. Brushing your teeth is the opposite of Pavlov's dog in the theory of operant conditioning. Brushing your teeth is a signal to your brain that you're done eating, and it's time to do something else. Not brushing your teeth leaves the idea open to you eating more. On the other hand, once you brush your teeth, it can feel like a nuisance to repeat it for the sake of nibbling on something.

245. Follow the Mediterranean Diet (MD)

Following the eating habits of people who live in the Mediterranean will reduce inflammation, increase weight loss, enhance heart health, and promote better blood sugar control. The style of eating encourages nutritious foods like fruits, vegetables, whole grains, and healthy fats while limiting processed ingredients and added sugar.

246. Eat with a Friend, so You Take Time to Chat During Your Meals

It takes 20 minutes for your stomach to signal to your brain that you're full. Therefore fast food, aside from being full of unhealthy additives, is made to be eaten as quickly as possible. Rushing through meals can cause you to overeat. One of the things I've always admired and appreciated was how people in Italy or France sit, eat, and chat for prolonged periods. As an American from a fast-paced city, this seemed like a luxury and reason enough to move to Europe, where people have a much greater appreciation of mealtime as a time to socialize and enjoy someone's company. Extend your meal times to at least 20 minutes by talking and visiting with family and friends while you eat.

247. Mindful Eating

Mindful eating is based on the Buddhist concept of mindfulness. Mindfulness is a type of meditation that helps you recognize and deal with your emotions and physical sensations. It's used to treat many health conditions, including psychological disorders and food-related behaviors

Mindful eating can help reduce food cravings and improve portion control. Using mindfulness, you can reach a state of full attention to your cravings, experiences, and physical cues when eating. Begin by avoiding distractions while eating, including computers, cell phones, televisions, and reading materials. People who eat while distracted can eat 10-25% more per meal, causing significant weight gain over time. Keeping your mind engaged while eating can prevent satiety cues from instructing your brain that you've had your fill. Instead, eat sitting comfortably at a table, concentrating on the taste of the food, and recognizing when you feel full.

Mindful eating can help you eat slower and help you manage your weight easier.

Mindful eating techniques:

- Eat slowly and without distractions.
- Pay attention to your hunger cues and stop when full.
- Be aware of real hunger and non-hunger causes of eating
- Engage all of your senses by noticing flavors, colors, sounds, smells, and textures.
- Deal with anxiety and guilt about food
- Eat to maintain health and not for fun
- Be aware of foods effects on your feelings and body

Taking these steps will help you appreciate your food and replace automatic thoughts and reactions with healthier responses.

248. Eating Together as a Family

Eating healthy can be lonely, especially when you try something new alone. But when you eat healthily together, you're much more likely to continue healthy eating habits longer. Home-cooked meals tend to be lower in fat, calories, and sugar than fast food. Learning to eat together as a family teaches children how to develop healthy eating habits.

W. Hacks for Snacks

249. Chew Gum

Chewing gum can be useful for overcoming cigarette cravings, improving your memory, and losing weight. Chewing gum can help promote weight loss, control cravings, and manage hunger. Sugar-free gum is best because it usually has less than five calories per piece, compared to ten calories for regular gum. Diet plans like Jenny Craig, Weight Watchers, and the American Diabetes Association consider sugar-free gum a fat free food because you burn more calories chewing it than what it contains.

Researchers have shown that people who chew gum consumed 68 fewer calories, satisfy cravings, reduce stress, and resist fattening treats. Gum chewers also burned about 5% more calories than non-gum chewers per day.

Another benefit is that some people have a psychological as well as a sensory need for oral stimulation. A stick of gum is a good substitute for something much higher in calories like chips or a doughnut.

Try gum when you have the desire to eat a snack between meals, during a movie instead of mindless snacking while watching TV or at a party. Keep some available when you get an unhealthy craving or while you cook to prevent nibbling.

Chewing gum, however, can also lead to tooth decay and erosion, especially when sweetened with sugar, which feeds the "bad" bacteria in your mouth, damaging your teeth. Chewing sugar-free gum is better when it comes to your dental health.

250. Eat Fillers

Before each meal eat a large salad, nuts, fruit, air-popped popcorn, whipped potatoes, or broth-based soup to help you get full faster, reduce calories, and lose weight. Choose foods that are full of fiber, air, or water.

251. Air Popped Corn

Most people love popcorn, especially during a movie, but movie popcorn is very high in calories and unhealthy chemicals. Try popping corn prepared in an air popper. Air popping helps make popcorn a high-fiber, low-calorie, whole-grain, and antioxidant-rich snack food. Ditch the butter, and sprinkle some salt and pepper, red pepper flakes, olive oil, cinnamon, or cocoa powder.

Three cups of air-popped popcorn have only 1 gram of fat, 93 calories, and almost 4 grams of fiber.

252. Emergency Late Night Snack

If it's late at night or outside of your eating window and you're starving, have a snack. Don't go to bed hungry, or you'll have a hard time sleeping, and you'll be hungrier the next day. Eating the right type of snack can boost your metabolism and increase weight loss. The ideal late-night snack is a glass of soy milk or cow's milk. Both are high in protein, and rich in tryptophan. Tryptophan is the precursor to serotonin in your brain. Theoretically, if you consume enough tryptophan, your brain will produce more serotonin a few hours later, which will make you relax and improve sleep. Soy milk has the added benefit of inducing a natural sedative effect by enhancing the body's melatonin levels and reducing the time needed to sleep.

If you feel the need to eat something substantial, eat a carbohydrate with a healthy fat such as pear slices and almond butter, celery with guacamole, and strawberries with heavy cream. All can help keep your blood sugar stable, so glucagon, a fat-burning hormone, can help you lose weight.

253. Advertise our Snacks

Eat whatever you like, but before doing so, yell out loud, "I'm not hungry, but I'm going to eat this anyway." This helps break negative eating behaviors by reminding yourself you can eat it, and I recognize that it's bad for you. By practicing this, you can lose around 2 pounds a month, but more importantly, it helps curb negative eating behaviors.

254. Eat Healthy Snacks

The size of snacks has increased over time, resulting in one-third of people's daily calorie consumption coming from snacks. This is an opportunity to choose healthy snacks to decrease the number of calories that people eat during meals and increase fullness. Eat snacks that center around fruits and vegetables and add some protein with each snack so you stay fuller longer.

Healthful snack options:

Apple slices with string cheese, orange with almonds, celery sticks with peanut butter, unflavored yogurt with berries and granola, carrots with hummus are examples of healthy snacks.

Mix and match high-fiber fruits, such as apples, strawberries, bananas, raspberries, and oranges, mangos, dried prunes, or dates with unsalted, unflavored nuts, including almonds, pistachios, or walnuts.

255. Nutrition Bars

Energy bars are high in carbs and sugar to give you a quick boost and prolonged endurance during activities. Protein bars are higher in protein content and are best used as meal replacements when on the go. Both are known as nutritional bars.

Nutritional bars are a popular snack food designed to be a convenient source of nutrition for curbing the appetite, fueling a workout, or supporting muscle repair after exercise. Because of their compact size and nutrient density, they can be great for a busy and active lifestyle. However, nutrition bars vary widely between brands, flavors, and some can be bad for your health. Nutritional bars contain 5-10 grams of fat and fiber, 25-35 grams of carbs, 10-40 grams of protein, 150-400 calories, and micronutrients, such as calcium, iron, magnesium, potassium, phosphorus, vitamin E, and B vitamins. Energy bars tend to be higher in carbs and lower in protein, while protein bars are the exact opposite.

Unfortunately, most nutritional bars are high in sugar and artificial sweeteners like high fructose corn syrup, which adds excess fructose to your diet and can increase your risk of fatty liver, obesity, and diabetes when consumed in high amounts. Lower quality bars can be as unhealthy as a candy bar, high in calories up to 400 calories, and can help promote obesity rather than cut calories. Unhealthy bars may also have unhealthy and fattening fats from highly processed plant oils such as palm, canola, peanut, or soybean oil.

Higher quality bars are made with dates, stevia, dried fruit, nuts and seeds, and whole grains like oats or quinoa. The protein can come from dairy proteins like casein and whey, eggs, soy, pea, brown rice, or nuts and seeds as a primary protein source.

Good quality nutritional bars can be useful for keeping you satiated when you're on the run and need something nutritious. Keep them close by to help curb your appetite and help prevent overeating.

Nutritional bars can also vary substantially in cost, and some of the most costly ones are not worth the high expense. Generally, nutritional bars with short ingredient lists that primarily use whole foods rather than highly processed ingredients and minimal to no added sugar are the best.

Another suggestion is to pack healthy foods as an alternative to nutritional bars, which tend to be highly processed, regardless of quality.

Healthy nutritional bar alternatives include;

- raw nuts and seeds

- hard-boiled eggs
- unsweetened yogurt
- nut and seed butter
- dairy or high-protein non-dairy milk
- tofu and tempeh
- cottage cheese
- beans and lentils
- certain whole grains
- seitan
- lean meats and fish
- cheese.

X. Travel

256. Jet Lag

Studies show that moving into different time zones, can cause you to eat more erratically, gain weight, and develop diabetes-related metabolic issues. Traveling and the subsequent change in our circadian rhythm changes our gut microbe growth in a way that encourages metabolic diseases. A change in our sleep-wake cycle can cause the replacement of our beneficial gut flora by bacteria that can cause obesity and metabolic syndrome. Because the bacteria in your stomach are not exposed directly to light, they adjust their circadian cycle to our mealtimes.

To help mitigate some of the weight gains, eat lots of fiber-rich snacks, stick to your regular meal times, and keep your eating habits as routine as possible.

257. Be Aware of the Effects of Living in a Northern Latitude

Living up north can affect the makeup of your gut bacteria and the amount of vitamin D you get in your body resulting in increased weight gain. Living in northern latitudes encourages the growth of Firmicutes microbes, which have been linked to weight gain while decreasing the number of bacteria linked with slim body types called Bacteroidetes. Research shows that the number of Firmicutes increases with latitude, and the number of Bacteroidetes decreases with latitude. To help ensure a healthy gut, consume fermented and probiotic-rich foods, both of which encourage the growth of healthy gut bacteria.

Starting in September, people who live in the northern hemisphere get less sunshine as the winter months begin, the days are shorter, and there is less sunshine. The skin uses ultraviolet B (UVB) sunlight to photolyze provitamin D3 to previtamin D3. The hormone is then converted into the active form of the vitamin by the liver and kidneys. Lower Vitamin D levels often mean lower calcium levels, and lower calcium levels will result in diminished weight loss.

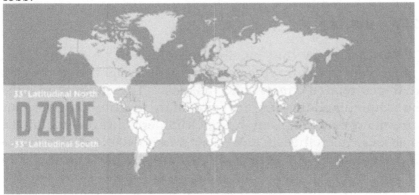

Your skin produces little if any vitamin D from the sun at latitudes above 33 degrees north (in the grey shaded area of the United States) or below 33 degrees south of the equator. Except for the summer months. Therefore, people who live in these areas are at higher risk for vitamin D deficiency.

258. Eat Locally Grown

The sooner you eat harvested fruits and vegetables, the more nutritious the food will be. Farmers pick their locally grown produce within 24 hours of selling them at farmer's markets. Imported produce is picked green so that it will last while it travels, sits in a distribution center, then arrives at your store, thus reducing the nutrient value, since most plants produce most of their nutrients during the final stages of ripening on the vine or branch. Therefore the fruit or vegetable may look the same, but the flavor and nutrient value will often be much lower. Your neighborhood farmer's market is an excellent place to buy fresh fruits and veggies.

The walk around the market is a good exercise, and it keeps you engaged with what you're eating, helping you make the most of your nutritionally-minded outing and exposing you to a variety of healthy foods. It also cuts down on the exposure and temptation of buying processed foods.

Local food has a shorter journey between harvest and your table, so it's good for the environment. When thinking about what's best for you to eat, consider what is best for the planet as well. Not consuming foods that have been flown or boated in from long distances will help reduce the carbon footprint of what you're eating and ensure its nutritional value. The money spent on food grown in your community gets reinvested with businesses and services in your town.

Locally grown food is safer, as the more steps there are between you and your food source, the higher the probability of contamination. Food that is grown and transported from distant locations can have food safety issues during harvesting, washing, shipping, and delivery. Local producers can tell you how the food was planted, grown, and harvested. Investing time in buying good food and learning about healthy eating will help you eat better as your nutritional intelligence increases.

Y. Supplements

We can get most of the nutrients from the food we eat without taking supplements with the exception of vitamin B12 and vitamin D. B12 because most things are over sanitized, and we don't eat enough beneficial dirt and vitamin D because we don't get enough sunlight. However, most people don't eat a balanced diet and end up with vitamin deficiencies.

The supplement industry is a 40-billion-dollar industry a year, and they have a lot of money to market a variety of products. Most of the products have inconsequential effects. Supplements are made by very few companies that sell their raw materials to other companies to put their brand on them. For example, a generic bottle of vitamin D can cost $5.00, while a name-brand bottle of the same vitamin bought from the same supplier can cost $40.00. The only difference is the company logo stamped on the bottle. Therefore, it's very unlikely that you'd get any additional benefits from paying more for name-brand supplements. When scientists measure vitamins in the blood, they find the levels are the same whether the person was taking a name brand or a generic brand.

Studies show the average American diet is deficient in several essential nutrients, including calcium, potassium, magnesium, and vitamins A, C, and D. Check out the National Institutes of Health (NIH), and National Center for Complementary and Integrative Health (NCCIH) websites for the latest research and recommendations on supplements.

Nutrient	How Much to Take	Don't Exceed
Calcium	1,000-1,2000 mg	2,000 mg
Folate	400 mcg	1,000 mcg
Iron	8 mg	45 mg

Vitamin A	700 mcg	3,000 mcg
Vitamin B6	1.5 mg	100 mg
Vitamin B12	2.4 mcg	Not established
Vitamin C	75 mg	2,000 mg
Vitamin D	600-800 IU	4,000 IU
Vitamin E	15 mg	1,000 mg

259. Vitamin D

Vitamin D is vital to immune function, bone growth, weight management, and multiple other body functions. Vitamin D is primarily made in your skin when exposed to sunlight. However, it can also be absorbed from the foods you eat and through supplementation. Foods that contain vitamin D include fatty fish, egg yolks, certain mushrooms, and fortified dairy products. Animal and human studies suggest that people who take a combination of vitamin D, vitamin K, and calcium lose two times more fat than others who don't. The three supplements have a synergistic effect that is beneficial for bone and cardiovascular health.

Over 42% of Americans are deficient in vitamin D, mostly due to working indoors. In ideal conditions, 10-15 minutes of sunlight on your arms and legs a few times a week can help you produce all of the vitamin D you need. However, ideal conditions are affected by the time of day, the season, location, cloud cover, and even pollution that can block the amount of UVB that reaches your skin. The more skin that is exposed, the more vitamin D your body will produce. Production of vitamin D is influenced by skin color (African Americans produce about half as much vitamin D as white Americans), and people age 65 and over generate only one-fourth as much vitamin D as people in their 20s.

The effects of sunscreen on vitamin D production is

minimal.

Sunscreen prevents sunburn by blocking UVB light. However, few people put on enough sunscreen to block all UVB light, or they use sunscreen irregularly.

260. Omega Fatty Acids

Fish oil derived from fatty fish like anchovies, mackerel, salmon, and cod is one of the world's most popular dietary supplements. Its health benefits come from two types of omega-3 fatty acids, docosahexaenoic acid (DHA) and eicosapentaenoic acid (EPA). Research shows that both have multiple health benefits, including improving weight loss, heart and brain health. The crustacean krill is also used to produce omega-3-fatty acid supplements and is better than fish oil. However, neither is sustainable, and due to environmental pollution, virtually all fish have unsafe levels of mercury and other toxins. Therefore their benefits may be outweighed by their toxicity. Although not as potent, you can use plant-based sources such as chia seeds, brussel sprouts, algal oil, hemp seed, walnuts, flaxseeds, and perilla oil.

261. Eat Dirt

Geophagy, the practice of eating soil, has been practiced for thousands of years to treat a variety of health problems. Consuming as little as 500 milligrams of dirt a day on produce could increase weight loss.

Eighty percent of people don't get enough B vitamins in their diet due to the modern sanitization of food. Over washing produce removes all of the dirt and destroys beneficial microorganisms. Soil-based organisms help keep your gut healthy and strengthen your immune response by feeding cells in the colon and liver, and killing harmful bacteria. Small amounts of dirt typically found on fruits and veggies from farmer's markets, where produce is not usually over-washed, is used by your body to make B-vitamins. B-vitamins and healthy intestinal bacteria are vital to weight loss. Grow some of your own produce or buy from farmer's markets, where food not only has soil, the food is fresher, and has higher nutritional content.

262. Aloe Vera.

Aloe vera juice is rich in B vitamins, C, E, and multiple minerals (calcium, copper, chromium, sodium, selenium, magnesium, potassium, manganese, and zinc). Aloe vera promotes weight loss by boosting your metabolism, increasing blood sugar control, improving digestion, and reducing inflammation in your body. This translates to a healthy digestive system, efficient processing of food, and detoxification which aids in losing weight

The gel inside of the leaves of the aloe vera plant should be removed and added to homemade smoothies, salads, soups, salsas, and stir-fries.

263. Apple Cider Vinegar

Apple cider vinegar is made by cutting up apples and combining them with yeast to convert their sugar into alcohol. The alcohol is then fermented into acetic acid using bacteria. The acetic acid is anti-inflammatory, lowers blood sugar, decreases insulin levels, burns fat, suppresses appetite, and reduces fat storage. Unfiltered apple cider vinegar has the cloudy "mother" on the bottom of the bottle. Mother is clusters of bacteria that have more gut-boosting benefits than the filtered vinegar. Adding apple cider vinegar to your diet can benefit blood sugar, insulin sensitivity, polycystic ovary syndrome (PCOS) symptoms, and cholesterol. Vinegar also fights bacteria and viruses.

Studies show that adding 1- 2 tablespoons of apple cider vinegar to your diet a day can help you lose around 0.9-1.2 pounds per month. Mix with juice or water and drink.

264. Creatine

Creatine is found naturally in muscle cells. Creatine supplements give you more energy, promote muscle growth, and facilitate weight loss. Creatine causes your muscle cells to store more water, which causes your muscles to look bigger. It also gives you more energy and strength to do more work during activities. Your muscles will get stronger and more prominent from this increased intensity.

Creatine is an effective supplement with powerful benefits for both athletic performance and health. It may boost brain function, fight certain neurological diseases, improve exercise performance, and accelerate muscle growth.

265. Resistant Starch

Most of the carbohydrates in the food we eat are starches. Starches are long chains of glucose found in grains, potatoes, and other foods. A portion of some starches is resistant starch, and it passes through your digestive tract undigested. It functions like soluble fiber, and it improves insulin sensitivity, causes weight loss, lowers blood sugar levels, reduces appetite, and improves digestion.

You can add resistive starches to your diet, by eating foods high in resistant starch such as raw potatoes, or cooked and cooled potatoes, green bananas, plantains, cashews, raw oats, cooked then cooled rice, barley, or legumes (black beans, navy beans, northern beans, black-eyed peas, peas, and lentils). Otherwise, take dry potato starch powder as a supplement.

Resistant starch is effective because it functions like soluble, fermentable fiber. It moves through your stomach and small intestine undigested, then reaching your colon, where it feeds your healthy bacteria. Resistant starch improves your health by feeding and growing the population of friendly bacteria in your intestines, where the bacteria use the resistive starch to produce short-chain fatty acids like butyrate.

Butyrate feeds the cells in your colon, which aids in reducing the pH level, reducing inflammation, increasing the absorption of minerals, lowering your risk of colorectal cancer, and aids in various digestive disorders. These include ulcerative colitis, Crohn's disease, constipation, diverticulitis, and diarrhea.

Adding a supplement like potato starch to your meals can increase feelings of fullness and help you eat fewer calories. It tastes bland, so you can sprinkle it on your food or mix into beverages without noticing it. Add about four tablespoons of potato starch to your meals throughout the day, start slowly and build slowly or you can cause flatulence and upset your stomach. Don't bother taking excess amounts as it will merely pass through your body when you reach 50-60 grams per day (4 teaspoons is 32 grams of starch). It'll take 2-4 weeks for the production of short-chain fatty acids to increase and for you to notice all the benefits.

266. Probiotics

Probiotics are beneficial bacteria that supplement bacteria in your intestines. Humans rely on bacteria for digestion and general health, while bacteria in the intestines rely on the host to provide them with fiber as food. A healthy gut is linked to optimal brain function, healthy weight, and mood. Other benefits provided by bacteria include: energy for the gut wall and liver cells, production of anti-cancer fatty acids, and maintaining body weight. Overeating sugar, meats, or taking pharmaceuticals can decrease your good bacteria and cause health problems. Probiotics can be introduced naturally by eating fermented foods, including sauerkraut, kefir, yogurt, miso, kombucha, tempeh, and kimchi.

Your body processes more than 25 tons of food over a lifetime, placing your gut on the frontline of pollution control. Maintaining healthy intestinal bacteria will allow it to filter the toxins found in the air, water, and food we consume. People who are overweight tend to have more bad bacteria in their gut. Consuming probiotic supplements will keep the gut flora healthy and strong.

Your body has hundreds of different species of bacteria in your intestines. The bacteria in your intestines (gut bacteria) outnumber the body's cells 10 to 1. Therefore, the food you eat feeds only 10% of your cells. Fermentable fibers, and resistant starches feed the other 90% (gut bacteria).

267. Chitosan

Chitosan is a dietary supplement made from chitin, which comes from the shells of crab, shrimp, and lobsters. It is believed that chitosan can fight fat absorption and work as a natural weight loss aid. However, not much research has been conducted to support the weight loss benefits of chitosan.

268. Meratrim

Meratrim is a supplement made of two plant extracts that change the metabolism of fat cells. The supplement makes it harder for fat cells to multiply, decreases the amount of fat absorbed from the bloodstream, and helps cells burn stored fat. On average, people lose 1.4 pounds a week, and have reduced blood sugar, cholesterol, and triglycerides. No known side effects have been found. The US National Institute of health studied meratrim and found it to be effective as a weight loss supplement.

269. Glucomannan

Glucomannan is a fiber supplement made from the roots of the elephant yam, also known as konjac. Glucomannan absorbs water and becomes gelatinous, causing it to sit in your gut and make you feel full so you eat less. On average, people lose 2 pounds a week using this supplement.

Glucomannan also feeds friendly bacteria in the intestine, lowers blood sugar, blood cholesterol, and triglycerides, and is effective against constipation. However, It can cause bloating, flatulence, and soft stools.

270. Hydroxycut

Hydroxycut is one of the most popular weight loss supplements in the world. It's made of several ingredients, including caffeine and plant extracts. People who use Hydroxycut lose around 1.5 pounds per week. However, if you're caffeine sensitive, you may experience anxiety, nausea, jitteriness, tremors, diarrhea, or irritability.

271. L-Tyrosine

If you're having difficulty getting rid of sugar cravings, try the amino acid l-tyrosine. It is used by your body to build proteins and reduce hunger for sweets by signaling to the brain to release the neurotransmitters dopamine (the feel-good hormone) and norepinephrine. Tyrosine can be found naturally in milk, some cheeses (Parmesan, Romano, Gruyère, and Swiss) eggs, spirulina, sesame seeds, beef, and bacon. Increasing tyrosine has been linked to a reduction in belly fat.

272. L-Glutamine

Glutamine is an amino acid that helps reduce and eliminate sugar cravings by helping to steady blood sugar. It gives you more energy, keeps weight off, accelerates weight loss, and maintains muscle mass. Add 500 milligrams of l-glutamine three times a day to meals, and a quarter teaspoon when you feel a sugar craving.

273. Folate

Folate is one of the B-vitamins and is needed to make red and white blood cells in the bone marrow, convert carbohydrates into energy, and produce DNA and RNA. People with the highest folate levels lose about 8.5 times more weight when dieting than those with the lowest levels of folate. Higher dietary folate intake also reduces breast cancer risk. Some foods that are high in folate include spinach, asparagus, papaya, and watercress. Watercress is high in folate and stimulates weight loss.

274. Gelatin

Gelatin is a protein product made from collagen. Research has shown that gelatin can improve joint health, brain function, slow cancer growth, promote sleep, improve skin and hair appearance, and facilitate weight loss. Gelatin is made by boiling animal skin, bones, tendons, and ligaments of mammals in water and extracting collagen. It can be eaten as bone broth, used in food, or taken as a supplement. Gelatin is the richest food source of the amino acid glycine. Gelatin is 98-99% protein, and the remaining 1–2% is water and small amounts of vitamins and minerals. It is abundant in these amino acids:

Glycine: 27%

Proline: 16%

Valine: 14%

Hydroxyproline: 14%

Glutamic acid: 11%

Amino acid composition varies depending on the method of preparation and the type of animal tissue used.

Gelatin is fat and carb-free and helps you lose weight. Studies show that eating gelatin increases hormones that reduce appetite and increases feelings of fullness. Gelatin expands in your stomach, reducing hunger by up to 44%. Add one to two tablespoons a day to coffee, juice, desserts, shakes, or meals for optimal results.

275. Chlorella

Chlorella is an ancient life form that is virtually unchanged for over 2 billion years. Studies show that chlorella reduces cravings due to its high nutritional content. Chlorella is an excellent source of many essential nutrients such as protein, beta carotene, nucleic acids (DNA and RNA), and has more chlorophyll than any other food. Chlorella is also high in gamma-linolenic acid (GLA), the crucial fatty acid that is often deficient due to dietary imbalances. GLA helps stabilize your endocrine system, restoring hormone health, normalizing insulin activity, balancing blood sugar levels, and reducing cravings.

Additionally, chlorella is 50-60% protein, low in calories, a complete food nutritionally, a rich source of vitamins, stimulates red blood cell production and arterial dilation, muscle growth, muscle tissue oxygen, improved metabolism, and respiration. For these reasons, chlorella is used in muscle-building and weight-loss supplements. Chlorella is also high in iodine, which is essential in treating thyroid imbalances, often an issue in weight problems.

Overweight and obese people are often malnourished. Supplying them with complete nutrition helps relieve intense food cravings. Eating chlorella will reduce the cravings of irregular food intake, improve the hunger cycle, and decrease refined food consumption. The essential nutrients in chlorella can reverse degenerative diseases by correcting and balancing nutritional deficits to restore optimal cellular and tissue function.

Chlorella regulates the digestive system, a problem associated with obesity and linked to the accumulation of toxic chemicals in the digestive system. It also binds with toxic substances such as mercury, making it easier for the body to remove them from the body. Chlorella is a probiotic that promotes the production of healthy bacterial flora throughout the digestive system. Chlorella is rich in fiber resulting in increased feelings of fullness at mealtimes and better food elimination.

Research shows that chlorella blocks fat cell production and shrinks existing ones. Preventing baby fat cells from maturing and becoming fat-storing cells when a person overeats. Chlorella promotes weight loss by controlling gene expression to produce reductions in body fat percentages, total circulating cholesterol, and fasting glucose levels.

Mix powdered chlorella into drinks, chew on tablets at the end of meals and reduce the desire to eat sweets, preventing blood sugar rushes and associated cravings.

276. Eliminate Unnecessary Pharmaceuticals

One of the most common questions I get from patients is why they've never had to take a medication before, and now that they're in the hospital, they have to take twenty or more pills a day? The answer is because most Americans are overprescribed. Americans are 5% of the world population but use over 75% of the world's pharmaceuticals. Seventy percent of Americans take on average ten pills a day.

One of the outcomes of taking so many medications is nonalcoholic fatty liver disease (NAFLD). Your liver is the largest organ inside your body. It helps your body store energy, digest food, and remove toxins. Fatty liver disease is a condition in which fat builds up in your liver and decreases the liver's ability to function. Poor diet, overconsumption of medications, environmental toxins, and disease are all causes of fatty liver disease.

Fatty liver disease, in turn, can cause hormonal imbalance, overall poor health, and weight gain. Speak to your physician about fatty liver tests and reducing the number of prescription and nonprescription medications you take to decrease your liver's workload and increase its efficiency.

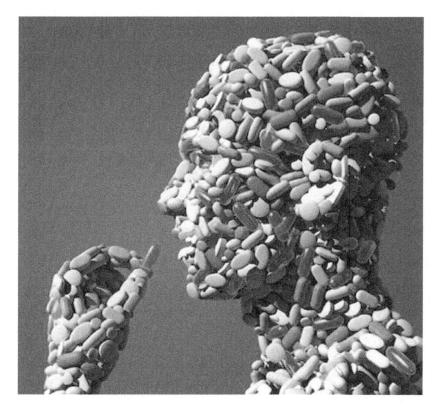

277. Melatonin

Sleep deprivation can interfere with body function, decrease energy levels, cause weight gain, and decrease overall fitness. If you have issues sleeping, melatonin is a naturally occurring hormone in your body that can be taken as a supplement to improve sleep. Melatonin is safe, does not cause a hangover effect, or have a diminished response over time (habituation), unlike pharmaceutical sleep medications that can cause dependence and harm your body.

The pineal gland secretes melatonin in the brain to help regulate our circadian rhythm. The circadian rhythm is your body's internal clock and controls your sleep-wake cycle. Circadian rhythms are optimal when we have regular sleep habits and are affected by sunrise and sunset. Darkness stimulates our brain's melatonin release, which causes sleepiness. Melatonin levels then peak in the middle of the night while we're sleeping, and as the sun rises, melatonin levels drop, which signals the body to wake up.

Melatonin is the primary hormone regulating our circadian rhythm, which is why it's important to address imbalances in the hormone if you have sleep problems. Melatonin also affects leptin and adiponectin, as well as insulin levels. These hormones help regulate fat burning, glucose regulation, and speed up your metabolism. Research shows that people who supplemented with melatonin showed decreased fat mass by 7%, increased lean mass by 2.9%, and adiponectin levels increased by 21%. Recommended melatonin doses are from 0.5 mg up to 3 mg, which are adequate to promote sleep or treat jet lag.

278. Matcha Powder

Matcha comes from the Camellia sinensis plant, like green tea. However, farmers grow matcha differently by covering their tea plants 20–30 days before harvest to avoid direct sunlight. The process gives the plant a dark green hue, increases chlorophyll and amino acid content.

Matcha contains all the nutrients from the entire green tea leaf, which results in a higher amount of caffeine and antioxidants than typically found in green tea. In addition, matcha is simple to prepare by mixing in cold or hot water or simply incorporating it effortlessly into your diet.

Six benefits of Matcha

1. Helps you Lose Weight

Look at any weight loss supplement, and most likely, "green tea extract" will be listed in the ingredients. Matcha speeds up your metabolism, increases energy expenditure, and boosts fat burning.

During moderate exercise, taking green tea extract increases fat burning by 17% and overall fat burning for 24 hours.

2. Loaded with Antioxidants

Matcha is rich in catechins, a powerful antioxidant that helps neutralize free radicals, harmful compounds that damage cells and cause chronic disease. The catechins in matcha are up to 137 times greater than in other types of green tea.

3. Boosts Brain Function

Research shows that matcha caused improvements in attention, reaction time, and memory. In addition, consuming 2 grams of green tea powder daily for two months helps improve brain function, especially in older people.

One-half teaspoon (about 1 gram) of matcha powder contains 35 mg of caffeine. Studies have linked caffeine consumption to improved brain function, faster reaction times, increased attention, and enhanced memory.

Matcha is also high in the amino acid L-theanine, which improves the effects of caffeine, helping prevent energy crashes, and increasing alertness. L-theanine also increases alpha wave activity in the brain, which induces relaxation and decreases stress levels.

4. Protects the Liver

Studies show that matcha prevents liver damage and decreases the risk of liver disease.

5. Prevents Cancer

Matcha green tea extract decreased tumor size and slowed the growth of breast cancer cells in studies. In addition, matcha is high in epigallocatechin-3-gallate (EGCG), a type of catechin with potent anti-cancer properties, and is effective against skin, prostate, lung, and liver cancers.

6. Promotes Heart Health

Heart disease is the number one killer worldwide of people over 35, accounting for an estimated one-third of all deaths. Matcha reduces total and "bad" LDL cholesterol and triglycerides and prevents the oxidation of LDL cholesterol. Drinking green tea reduces your risk of stroke and heart disease.

279. Glycine

Glycine is an amino acid used by your body to build proteins, grow and maintain tissue, and make essential substances, such as hormones and enzymes. Glycine is abundant in gelatin and can improve memory, attention and reduce schizophrenia and OCD symptoms. Glycine is a liver detoxifier and improves its ability to burn fat.

Your body needs glycine to make essential compounds, such as glutathione, creatine, and collagen. Glutathione is an antioxidant that helps protect your cells against oxidative damage caused by free radicals. Glycine is a vital component of creatine, a compound that provides your muscles with energy, improves bone health, and brain function. Glycine is the most bountiful amino acid in collagen, a structural protein with several health benefits, including for your skin, joints, and bones. Glycine promotes sleep and enhances your sleep quality through its calming effects on the brain and its ability to lower core body temperature. The amino acid also protects your liver from alcohol-induced damage and heart health. Glycine can decrease your risk for heart disease by preventing plaque build-up and by increasing your body's ability to use nitric oxide. Supplementing with glycine may improve impaired insulin utilization in type 2 diabetes. Glycine helps preserve muscle mass in wasting conditions, such as cancer, malnutrition, and burns.

Glycine is available as a dietary supplement in powder or capsule form. The powder dissolves easily in water and has a sweet taste. Due to its sweet taste, glycine powder is used as a sweetener for food and drinks.

Z. Increasing Activity Levels for Faster Weight Loss

280. Increase Non-Exercise Activity Thermogenesis (NEAT)

Calories are primarily burned in 3 ways:

1) Your resting metabolic rate (necessary body functions for life).
2) Digesting food
3) moving around (NEAT).

There are two types of activity thermogenesis:

- Exercise activity thermogenesis is calories burned doing an intentional activity (gym, going for a walk, swimming, jogging, etc.).

- Non-exercise activity thermogenesis (NEAT) is calories burned while completing our activities of daily living, including sleeping, eating, digesting food, walking the dog, paid work, everything that is not an intentional activity to lose weight.

Your job impacts how much NEAT results from your daily work. Construction workers, personal trainers, dance instructors, or bartenders are examples of occupations that have a high level of NEAT.

For people that work in offices or other sedentary jobs, they tend to have low levels of NEAT.

Going to the gym for an hour at the end of the day after sitting for eight hours at work behind a desk will not make up for the low levels of activity throughout the day. Increasing the number of small activities throughout the day will accumulate the calories burned and be much more beneficial to you than spending an hour at the gym. Depending on your occupation, your NEAT can vary by up to 2,000 calories a day, whereas an hour on the stationary bike only burns 300 to 400 calories.

Jobs are requiring less and less movement from people, therefore, your job has a massive impact on your daily activity level. Improved transportation, cellphones, video games, online shopping, and delivery services are helping expedite the trend towards less activity. Sitting is the new smoking, causing worldwide obesity. Don't focus solely on the food you eat; analyze your activity levels.

Plan activities every hour to increase your NEAT. Avoid sitting when possible, you can burn an average of 350 calories more per day by standing. Ten minutes of activity will speed up your metabolism, and the more you move, the more it speeds up. Increasing your NEAT will decrease the size of your waist, making you look younger. Keep in mind that after age 45, you lose about ½ pound of muscle per year. The calories that those muscles would have burned will now be stored as fat.

281. Five Strategies for Increasing NEAT

- **Do your chores**

Gardening, house cleaning, washing clothes, or washing your car, are all simple ways to boost your activity level.

- **Use the stairs**

When possible, avoid elevators or escalators and take the stairs, even if it's just for part of your journey. More of the benefits in #259.

- **Stand whenever possible**

Standing burns about 54 calories over a six-hour day, and over 1,000 calories a month by staying on your feet. Use a standing desk rather than sitting to complete office work. Standing also helps prevent back and neck pain from sitting too long.

- **Schedule movement breaks**

If you're going to participate in an activity that requires little movement such as watching television or working at a desk, include physical movement with the event every hour. For example, don't use your remote control when watching television. Get up to manually adjust the volume. At the office, get up and get a glass of water from a distant location, deliver messages in person, or just go on a 10-15 minute walk every few hours.

- **Do More of Your Errands**

Avoid some of the modern conveniences when possible. Walk instead of using scooters, buy your own groceries, shop in a store instead of buying online when time allows.

282. Increase the Frequency of Your Sex

During foreplay and intercourse, you'll experience increased heart rate, blood pressure, respiratory rate, and calories expended. On average, women burn off 69 calories, and men burn off 100 per sex session. The process known as the sexual-response cycle has multiple health benefits, including:

- Weight Loss
- Longer Life Span
- Lower Heart Attack Risk
- Reduced Prostate Cancer Risk
- Less Colds & Improved Immune System
- Lower Blood Pressure
- Looking Younger
- Improved Libido
- Improved Strength
- Improved Bladder Control (especially for women)
- Reduced pain
- Improved Fertilization for Pregnancy
- Improved Sleep
- Improved Cardiovascular Health
- Stress Relief

- Improved Intimacy and Relationships
- Improved Calorie Expenditure
- Boost Brainpower
- Strengthens Your Well-Being
- Builds Endurance

If you're having difficulty with erectile dysfunction, it's a sign that you're having circulatory problems. The smaller vessels in your body get clogged first, which means you may not be eating correctly. Eating meat does not make you more macho, it causes erectile dysfunction, blocks your arteries, and decreases your blood circulation. Plant-based diets are better for your sex life.

283. Take a Walk Outside

Walking outdoors not only burns calories, it also causes a sense of pleasure, enthusiasm, increases self-esteem, lowers rates of depression, tension, and fatigue. Improving your mental health and mood can lead to healthier food choices.

284. Gardening

Gardening is one of the most beneficial and relaxing options for increasing your activity level. People who garden are 11 to 16 pounds lighter than those who don't. If done regularly, you can get sunlight, fresh air, and lose weight without even being aware that you're doing it. Yard work such as raking, pruning, soil tilling, digging, planting, and weeding can burn up to 200 calories.

285. Have a Walking Meeting

Walking meetings are an excellent way to get work done, exercise, and get some fresh air. A walking meeting is a meeting held while taking a walk away from meeting rooms, coffee shops, or offices. Research shows that walking boosts creative output by about 60%, and you can quickly burn 150 calories in just 30 minutes by walking and talking.

286. Take a Hike

Hiking provides many health benefits, from the physical activity being out on the trail, to emotional and mental betterment that comes from being in nature.

Hiking is one of the best whole-body workouts.

The benefits of hiking include:

- Decreased stress levels, enhanced mental wellbeing, and improved mood
- Lower blood pressure
- Reduced risk for heart disease
- Lower cholesterol levels
- Improved cardiovascular health
- A decrease in respiratory problems
- Improved weight control
- Lower body fat
- Improved osteoarthritis outcomes
- Improved bone density
- Increases in flexibility and coordination
- Enhanced relationships with friends and family
- Better quality of life

Spending time in nature reduces stress, anxiety, boosts mood, and can lead to a lower risk of depression. Being outdoors taking in the sights, smells, and feelings of nature opens up your senses to your surroundings and improves your sensory perception.

Hiking with a friend, partner, neighbor, family member, or in a group is more fun and builds a healthy relationship.

Hiking also burns significantly more calories than walking. Walking burns approximately 300 calories per hour, while hiking burns over 450 calories per hour. You could burn even more calories on more strenuous hikes

287. Walk your Calls

Next time you get a phone call from someone, stand up

and start walking for the duration of the call instead of sitting down. You can burn 150 calories per 30 minute phone call.

288. Use Public Transportation

Using public transportation can help diminish your carbon footprint, avoid traffic, and help you lose weight. It's an excellent way to increase non-exercise activity thermogenesis (NEAT). Whether you walk a few blocks to the nearest bus stop, ride a bike, or hustle between transfers to different subway lines, you're sneaking in a little exercise here and there. These small amounts of activity can help you sleep better and improve your cardiovascular health.

Researchers have found that people who drive to work gain more weight than those who use public transportation. Commuting by car adds an average of 5.5 pounds to your body, whether you exercise or not. People who take public transportation to work are 27% less likely to have high blood pressure, 44% less likely to be overweight, and 34% less likely to have diabetes. If possible, consider leaving the car at home and biking, walking, or commuting to work using public transportation a few times per week.

289. Walk Faster

Whether you're walking to the restroom, your dog, or to your car, make those steps count by increasing their fat burning. Instead of merely strolling 3.1 mph, pick up the pace to 3.5 MPH to 4, you'll end up burning an extra 1,200 calories a month.

290. Kegel Exercises

If you sit for long periods during the day, Kegels have multiple benefits. By holding a small ball or a folded pillow between your thighs and squeezing, you can work your pelvic floor muscles. By applying thigh bands, you can strengthen your butt and thighs. Merely working on this while you work at your desk helps burn calories, improve circulation, help with incontinence, makes the female vagina firmer and tighter during intercourse, and assists with erectile dysfunction.

291. Intermittent Activity

For every hour of TV watched after age 25, you lose 22-minutes of average life expectancy. A person who spends an average of six hours per day watching TV can expect to live 4.8 years fewer than someone who does not.

To make watching TV healthier, increase your activity level by using commercials for activity breaks. During each break complete one activity, doing as many as you can. If you're watching a streaming service, take a break every 30 minutes and do five minutes of activity. Switch activities at each commercial segment, until you work the entire body. For example, push-ups, squats, reverse lunges, sit-ups, and jumping jacks. The movie segment becomes your recovery time.

292. Weigh yourself Down

Keep ankle weights and a weighted vest in your car so you can slip them on when you're running errands. Either one can easily be concealed under loose clothing.

You can use either one or both to maximize your workout. Weighted vests have an option to add additional weight as desired. For someone short on time, this is an excellent way to burn calories and build muscle.

293. Take-Two Minutes

No matter how busy you get during the day, you only need two and a half minutes to boost your metabolism and burn calories. Research has shown that people who did five 30-second bursts of max-effort activity such as jumping jacks, squats, running upstairs, or burpees, with a four-minute rest in between boosted their metabolism for the next 24-48 hours, and burned 200 extra calories that day.

294. Sit on a Therapy Ball

Sitting on a therapy ball instead of an office chair can help you burn calories and build your core muscles while you work. An exercise ball's instability requires the user to increase trunk muscle activation and thus increase core strength and improve posture. Try sitting on a sports ball for 30-minute increments during the day to burn an additional 100 calories a day which adds up to an extra 30,000 calories or about 8.5 pounds a year for 300 days of work.

295. Take the Stairs

Taking the stairs is surprisingly effective in helping people lose weight. When faced with either taking an elevator, escalator, or stairs, climbing stairs allows you to burn twice as many calories as walking. By climbing two flights (flight=10 steps) of stairs a day, a 150-pound person could lose about 6 pounds per year. If you climb four flights of stairs a day, you'd lose 12 pounds a year or a pound a month without going to the gym.

Stair climbing helps prevent a sedentary lifestyle, strengthen muscles, improve cardiovascular fitness, reduce stroke risk, and burn more calories than jogging. In a study conducted by the United States National Institute of Health, people 26–67 years old who climbed 1-6 flights of stairs spent on average 13.1 seconds to travel between each floor by stairs and 37.5 by elevators. People saved about 15 minutes a day taking the stairs versus the elevator.

Most participants self-reported that fatigue from climbing stairs did not impact their daily routine, and they could continue their duties without resting. Using the elevator usually involves extra time due to waiting for its arrival. The time of day and day of the week also impacts the amount of time spent waiting for the elevator. Taking the stairs instead of the elevator saves about 15 minutes each workday. This 3% savings per workday could translate into improved fitness and productivity.

296. Stretch

If you don't actively stretch, you'll lose 10% of your flexibility every ten years. Stretching at least three times a week will prevent falls, improve balance, relieve pain, tension, and improve circulation. Regular stretching will also make it easier for you to move and make your body feel good. When you feel good, you're more likely to move more often, burn more calories, and improve your chances of weight loss.

297. Don't Depend on Exercise to Compensate for a Lousy Diet

Generally, weight loss is 75% diet and 25% exercise. Many people think that they can exercise to make up for poor eating habits. However, if you're trying to lose weight, it's much more essential to manage what you eat versus trying to burn it off through exercise. Exercise helps keep you healthy, but it's not enough to counteract a bad diet.

Consider some of the most common lunch foods. A slice of pizza can contain over 1200 calories. A 150-pound person would have to swim for two hours to burn off one slice of pizza. A burger can have from 350- 900 calories, large order of french fries 450 calories, and a doughnut 350 calories.

In one hour of exercise, the same person would burn; 600 calories swimming, 400 calories walking, and 360 calories doing yoga.

Conclusion

A. Consider Exercise to Help with Weight Management

Some people think that because they go to the gym five times a week they're off the hook. However, the US Centers for Disease Control and Prevention (CDC) says that only 10 percent of adults who work out at gyms get enough exercise to keep weight off.

Although we do not promote exercise as a primary tool for losing weight, it does have many benefits and is part of a healthy lifestyle. The CDC recommends at least 30 minutes, five days a week of moderate-intensity activity, such as a brisk walk, to stay healthy. But, to maintain a stable weight over the long term, you'll need around 60 minutes on most days, according to the American Council on Exercise.

Getting started on a weight loss plan can be difficult, but when you do, you're five times more likely to succeed in your long-term weight-loss goals if you start by dropping pounds rapidly. You also have to have a reason to lose weight, think of a reason, and focus on that reason for your motivation.

Typically limiting calorie intake and increasing physical activity are the standard prescription for both losing weight, improving health, and preventing weight gain. However, weight loss due to calorie restriction is ineffective as it results in a decrease in total bodily energy expenditure. A drop in expenditure slows continued weight loss and can contribute to weight regain unless you continue cutting calorie intake.

Continuing to burn calories during weight loss, or increasing it after weight reduction, with a lower-carbohydrate, higher-fat diet, could help facilitate further weight loss and prevent weight regain. The mix of calories from carbohydrates or fats is a critical factor in maintaining healthy body weight.

Losing weight is the first obstacle to overcome when treating obesity. The second obstacle is maintaining that loss. Only gradual and sustained weight reduction through dietary changes can prevent the negative health consequences associated with obesity. However, maintaining significant weight loss is notoriously tricky. Therefore, lifestyle redesign, developing healthy strategies that facilitate maintenance of reduced body weight is critical for the effective long-term treatment of obesity. The suggestions in this book will give you a roadmap on how to proceed next in your weight loss journey.

Like Steve Jobs the founder of Apple once said, "Whichever stage in life we are at right now, with time, we will face the day when the curtain comes down. Treasure Love for your family, love for your spouse, love for your friends... Treat yourself well. Cherish others. Love the people God sent you, one day He'll need them back."

B. Sample Daily Weight Loss Routine

6:00 AM

1) Wake up early.
2) Weigh yourself and record your weight.
3) Open the curtains and fill your bedroom with sunlight.
4) Drink 16 ounces of lemon water.
5) Dress up to stretch and exercise.
6) Stretch

Yoga is an excellent option to use for its strengthening and simultaneous stretching components. Below is a sample yoga program for beginners for enhancing and maintaining mobility. Assuming each position for thirty seconds, each will allow you to complete a stretch routine in 3-5 minutes.

Complete four exercises in 3-5 minutes.

Jumping Jack: 40 reps two sets

Wall Push up: 25 reps two sets

Walking lunges: 20 reps each side two sets

Mountain climber: 20 reps each side two sets

Exercising first thing in the morning accelerates your metabolism the rest of the day, makes it easier to stick to the program, allows you to lose weight more quickly, and helps maintain a healthy weight. Working out before breakfast combats the effects of eating high-calorie, high-fat diets.

People who engage in exercise first thing in the morning are 75% more likely to do so every day, while only half of those who worked out later in the day maintained their fitness schedule. Early-morning exercise improves sleep quality, improves cognitive function, and helps you make better decisions.

7:00 AM

1) Taking a cold shower before meditation acts as a symbolic cleansing.
2) Mindfulness meditation while sitting out in the sun.
3) Pack your lunch and snacks for the day. Planning your food helps you eat healthier and take fewer calories. It also prevents binge eating.
4) Drink at least one glass of fluids.
5) Wear fitted clothing.

8:00 AM

1) Mix up Your Commute
   Research shows that walking, biking, or using public transportation lowers body weight and reduces the risk of weight gain.
2) Keep your iPhone with you all day, so you register your steps.
3) Always take the stairs and park your bike or car in the furthest parking spot.
4) Drink at least one glass of fluids.

9:00 AM

1) Drink at least one glass of fluids.
2) Sit on a therapy ball while working at your desk.
3) Go for a walk during phone calls whenever possible.

10:00 AM

1) Breakfast should be the largest meal of the day and high in protein.
2) Enjoy your meal with a friend.
3) Use a small red plate for your meal. Pack meals made at home in glass, avoid plastics.
4) Track your food and drink intake using an iPhone app or a notepad.
5) Take your supplements with your meal.
6) Brush your teeth.

7) Walk at least 5 minutes, delivering messages to coworkers instead of calling them.

11:00 AM

1) Drink at least one glass of fluids.
2) Walk to the restroom furthest from your desk.
3) Listen to classical music while working to help you relax.

12:00 PM

1) Go on a walking lunch break outside with a friend.
2) Tell funny stories and have fun.
3) Drink at least one glass of fluids.
4) Eat a snack.

1:00 PM

1) Drink at least one glass of fluids.
2) Take a walking meeting outside, if possible.

2:00 PM

1) Eat lunch with friends.
2) Use multiple small plates for your food.
3) Quench your meal by having a side salad with your hamburger.
4) Instead of eating the brownies for dessert, smell them.
5) Brush your teeth.

3:00 PM

1) Drink at least one glass of fluids.
2) Listen to music while working.
3) Work at a standing desk.
4) Chew gum.

4:00 PM

1) Drink at least one glass of fluids.
2) Exercise and eat a snack.

3) Got a craving for a Snickers Bar? Then drink some water, eat something healthy, and then have a small portion of the unhealthy food you crave. If you're having a sugar craving, eating some protein will help calm or get rid of the temptation.
4) Kegel exercises while you work at your desktop.

5:00 PM

1) Drink at least one glass of fluids.
2) Take a stretch break.
3) Organize your office.
4) Chew gum.

6:00 PM

1) Dinner with the family
2) Wash the dishes.
3) Brush your teeth.

7:00 PM

1) Drink at least one glass of fluids.
2) Go grocery shopping.
3) Read the labels of everything you buy. If you don't know what something is, google it.

8:00 PM

1) Drink at least one glass of fluids.
2) Relax in a bathtub or swimming pool with your partner.

9:00 PM

1) Drink at least one glass of fluids.
2) Power down and calm your body to prepare it for sleep.
3) Read a book, watch TV, or have sex.
4) Close the curtains to block out ambient light.

10:00 PM

1) Turn off all lights and sounds (occasionally listen to hypnosis for deep sleep and relaxation. Use a sleep mask, black-out curtains, and earplugs if necessary.
2) Rest 7-8 hours for most adults, getting adequate sleep will make tomorrow's 24 hours of weight loss easier.
3) Sample Eating Guide

C. Sample Eating Guide

7-day menu

This sample menu includes various nutrient, fiber, and protein-rich meals to help you reach your weight loss goals. Adjust portion sizes to your individual needs. If you exercise in the morning, adjust your first mealtime to eat within a half hour after your exercise, and adjust the rest of the hours on your eating schedule accordingly. For example, if you finish exercising at, 7 am you'll want to eat within a half hour of your workout, so you'd have your first meal at 7:30 am, and your last meal would be at 3:30 pm.

Monday

09:00 am Drink three glasses of water with matcha powder and lemon juice (adjust the amount of water depending on your body weight)

10:00 am Breakfast: overnight oats made with rolled oats, chia seeds, and soy milk, topped with fresh berries and pumpkin seeds.

11:00 am Drink three glasses of water

12:00 Snack: mixed raw nuts with dried prunes

01:00 Drink three glasses of water

02:00 Lunch: Egg sandwich made with Ezeqiel sprouted bread and coconut oil mayonnaise with fresh basil, tomato, and avocado salad.

03:00 Drink three glasses of water

04:00 Snack: mango-spinach, almond, and soymilk smoothie

05:00 Drink three glasses of water

06:00 Dinner: homemade cauliflower-crust pizza topped

with pesto, onions, mushrooms, olives, peppers, spinach, marinated chicken or tempeh, and extra virgin olive oil drizzled on top.

07:00 Drink three glasses of water

Tuesday

09:00 am Drink three glasses of water with matcha powder and lemon juice

10:00 Breakfast: smoothie made with baby greens, frozen cherries, banana, homemade protein powder, flax seeds, and soy milk

11:00 am Drink three glasses of water

12:00 Snack: Banana with peanut butter

01:00 Drink three glasses of water

02:00 Lunch: mixed green salad with cucumber, onion, tomato, sweet potato, olives, grilled salmon or chickpeas, and extra virgin olive oil

03:00 Drink three glasses of water

04:00 Snack: sliced apple with almond butter

05:00 Drink three glasses of water

6:00 Dinner: red lentil dahl served on a bed of baby spinach, buckwheat, and half an avocado

07:00 Drink three glasses of water

Wednesday

09:00 am Drink three glasses of water with matcha powder and lemon juice

10:00 Breakfast: Spanish omelet made with eggs, mushrooms, onions, and peppers, served with guacamole and salsa

11:00 am Drink three glasses of water

12:00 Snack: unflavored Greek yogurt with berries and granola

01:00 Drink three glasses of water

02:00 Lunch: Lentil soup and Greek salad made with tomatoes, cucumbers, onion, feta cheese, and olives and dressed with salt, pepper, Greek oregano, and extra virgin olive oil

03:00 Drink three glasses of water

04:00 Snack: homemade trail mix using your favorite raw unsalted nuts and unsweetened dried fruit

05:00 Drink three glasses of water

06:00 Dinner: chicken or veggie meatballs in a marinara sauce served with spaghetti squash with a side of mixed baby greens and topped with nutritional yeast or Parmesan cheese and extra virgin olive oil

07:00 Drink three glasses of water

Thursday

09:00 am Drink three glasses of water with matcha powder and lemon juice

10:00 Breakfast: plain Greek yogurt topped with fresh fruit and chopped walnuts

11:00 am Drink three glasses of water

12:00 Snack: carrots with hummus

01:00 Drink three glasses of water

02:00 Lunch: Baby greens salad topped with a poached egg or marinated seitan, dried cranberries, cherry tomatoes, whole-grain pita chips, balsamic vinaigrette, and extra virgin olive oil-based dressing

03:00 Drink three glasses of water

04:00 Snack: carrots, radishes, and jicama dipped in black bean spread

05:00 Drink three glasses of water

06:00 Dinner: beef or a veggie burger topped with lettuce, tomato, roasted peppers, caramelized onions, and pickles, served on an Ezekiel sprouted bun and coleslaw made with coconut oil mayonnaise and stevia on the side.

07:00 Drink three glasses of water

Friday

09:00 am Drink three glasses of water with matcha powder and lemon juice

10:00 Breakfast: breakfast salad made with spinach, walnuts, blueberries, coconut flakes, raspberry vinaigrette, and two hard-boiled eggs

11:00 am Drink three glasses of water

12:00 Snack: celery sticks with peanut butter

01:00 Drink three glasses of water

02:00 Lunch: homemade veggie spring rolls with tofu, dipped in peanut butter sauce and served with a side of raw veggies

03:00 Drink three glasses of water

04:00 Snack: burrito made with sprouted tortilla black beans, brown rice, and cottage cheese

05:00 Drink three glasses of water

06:00 Dinner: veggie chili served on a bed of greens and wild rice

07:00 Drink three glasses of water

Saturday

09:00 am Drink three glasses of water with matcha powder and lemon juice

10:00 Breakfast: pumpkin pancakes topped with Greek or plant-based yogurt, chopped nuts, and fresh berries

11:00 am Drink three glasses of water

12:00 Snack: Apple slices with string cheese

01:00 Drink three glasses of water

02:00 Lunch: tuna or chickpea salad, served atop mixed greens with sliced avocado, sliced apple, and walnuts

03:00 Drink three glasses of water

04:00 Snack: Dark chocolate with nut butter

05:00 Drink three glasses of water

06:00 Dinner: grilled salmon or tempeh, quinoa, and sautéed kale

07:00 Drink three glasses of water

Sunday

Have some fun learning to cook a new low-calorie recipe or trying out a new healthy restaurant. If you've been craving certain foods, drink some water, eat something healthy, and then have a small portion of the unhealthy food you crave. Try to quench your meals as much as possible. Enjoy, but keep your hard work in mind while you're eating your favorite foods.

Some folks recommend a cheat day, and it may be an option for some, however, having a cheat day is never a good idea for some people because food is a drug, and any cheating can cause a relapse into bad eating habits. Try reducing your cheat meals little by little and try to get accustomed to the new lifestyle you have designed for yourself. If you do have a cheat meal, keep it to 10-20% of your regular calorie intake.

My father was a butcher, and we grew up eating a lot of meat. One day while at a tailgate, I over ate at a BBQ, and my body told me I needed a break as I felt sluggish, tired, and heavy. So, I first started with a one-week vegetable juice fast. Then I decided to try not to eat meat for one week. After the week, I felt great and decided to go for a second week. After realizing how easy it was not eating meat for a second week, I decided to go for one month as a personal goal. That one-month marker came and went, and I just never thought about eating meat again, 16 years later, I'm still a vegetarian. For most people, the idea of never being able to eat or do something makes you want to do it more. It's like the forbidden fruit that Eve ate in the garden of Eden. With that in mind, I never say, "I can't eat meat," instead, I say, "Not right now." I leave the door open if I ever feel the absolute necessity to eat meat, then I would do it and not make a big deal about it. Knowing I can eat meat, makes things a lot easier for me to continue with my new way of life. Expending too much energy trying to avoid something that is all around you, is going to suck a lot of time and energy out of you, and eventually, you'll be too tired of fighting off the craving and give in.

In the many years that I have worked in drug rehabilitation, I have learned that addiction is a very potent obstacle to overcome. In fact, the majority of people who leave drug rehabilitation relapse back into drug use. Sometimes just one dose of your drug of choice can cause you to say, "Forget it, I already screwed up anyway," and go all out. Unfortunately, this is the story I've heard many times over the years from my patients who have suffered from drug addiction. Interestingly, I listened to the same stories coming from patients trying to lose weight, and the struggle can be even more challenging. Imagine if you had a cocaine addiction and were bombarded with advertisements from television, social media, radio, at stores, bus benches, social gatherings, work events, and even friends. It would be almost impossible to stop using when even the people you love and trust offer you your drug of choice day in and out. Add in people you trust and respect, such as celebrities and athletes pushing those same drugs on you, and it becomes an insane scenario.

To attain lasting and meaningful weight loss, we have to learn to live with the temptations around us while practicing lifestyle redesign to achieve our weight loss and health goals. Use this book to help you create habits and routines that are personally meaningful and health-promoting.

D. Top Ten General Rules for Eating Healthy

Rule #1 Don't drink your calories. Sugary and calorie-filled beverages do not register the same as solid food, so you could drink an entire meal worth of calories and then go on to eat a full meal. Change your lifestyle to start drinking water, coffee, teas, and to increase your fluid intake in general. Making this lifestyle choice is probably the easiest way to start losing weight immediately.

Rule #2 No commercial shakes, powders, bars, fried, or processed foods.

Rule #3 Quench foods when eating out or eating unhealthy foods. For example, swap a salad or vegetables in place of french fries or other high-calorie foods to help reduce the damage from the burger.

Rule #4 Eat as much as you like, until you're full, and stop. An easy rule to remember is to eat untill you're 80% full and stop. Please keep it simple by picking 3-4 meals and repeating them. People who go on low carbohydrate diets sometimes complain of low energy and give up because they don't eat enough calories. A 1/2 cup of white rice is 300 calories, while a 1/2 cup of spinach is 15 calories. Vegetables are not calorically dense, so you must add protein for caloric load, and to help you feel satisfied.

Rule #5 We should be eating a plant-based diet 90-95% of the time. If you're sick, you should be eating 100% plant-based.

Rule #6 Use a lifestyle redesign to figure out your "WHY" as to the purpose, reason, and benefits for losing weight. Once you start your new life, don't tease yourself with bad foods, and you'll be able to avoid most of the adverse health effects.

Rule #7 If you have an overwhelming desire to eat something, drink some water, eat something healthy, and then have a small portion of the unhealthy food you crave. Spiking caloric intake once in a while increases fat loss, ensuring that your metabolic rate doesn't slow down from extended caloric restriction which helps maintain calorie burning at a higher level. Therefore, occasionally eating something you're trying to reduce or eliminate from your diet can be useful. However, planning an entire "cheat day" is a poor way to forget and lose the taste for unhealthy foods. Remember that processed foods loaded with salt, sugar, and other addictive qualities will keep you coming back for more. The more often you're exposed to them, the harder it will be to reduce them from your diet and redesign your lifestyle. These foods are made in laboratories to keep you addicted and buy more. The longer you avoid them, the easier it will be to develop a new lifestyle and increase your enjoyment of healthy foods. Honestly, baked sweet potato fries will never taste as good as all the chemicals and stimulants in Doritos corn chips, but the longer I go without eating Doritos, the less I crave them or even want to eat them. I believe in making a long-term, sustainable lifestyle redesign, cheat as little as possible, and get used to a new skinnier person lifestyle.

Rule #8 Increase your activity level. The more active you are, the better your physical state will be, which helps improve your psychological state, which lends itself to having better overall health and happiness. The easiest way to increase your activity level is to start a physical hobby such as golf, gardening, martial arts, swimming, hiking, etc.

Rule #9 Instead of eating fast foods, eat more slow foods. Foods such as fruits, vegetables, and high fiber foods that are digested much slower and keep you full longer compared to fast foods.

Rule #10 Keep it simple. Weight-loss strategies have to be easy so that they can be picked up as new habits.

E. Top Ten Factors to Keep in Mind for Optimal Health

1) Friends

2) Self-confidence

3) Sunlight

4) Res

5) Diet

6) Happiness

7) Posture

8) Avoiding the use of alcohol, drugs and tobacco.

9) Have fun

10) Physical activity.

F. Top Books on Nutrition

1) The China Study

2) Conscious Eating

3) The Zone.

G. Top Ten Weight Loss iPhone Applications

1) iPhone Health

2) RunKeeper

3) Strava

4) Fitness Point

5) Fitocracy

6) Fitbit

7) C25K 5K Trainer

8) Nike Training Club

9) Fit Radio

10) 7 Minute Workout

H. Top 5 foods to Avoid

a. Processed, commercial, and BBQ meats.

b. Full-fat dairy including ice cream, butter, whole milk, and trans-fat-laden margarine (fake diary).

c. Fried, grilled, or broiled foods.

d. Soft drinks, sugar, fruit juices, and artificial sweeteners.

e. White flour products.

I. Top Weight Loss Websites

1) Loseit.com

2) Myfitnesspal.com

3) Fooducate.com

4) Sparkpeople.com

5) Supertracker.usda.gov

6) Calorieking.com

7) Fitday.com

8) Sparkpeople.com

9) Webmd.com

10) Cspinet.org

11) Nusi.org

12) Nutritionaction.com

13) Unscn.org

14) Medlineplus.org

15) Ncbi.nlm.nih.gov

16) MyFoodData.com

About the Author

Dr. Ernesto Martinez suffered a near-fatal assault that changed the direction of his life. The experience helped him acquire a greater moral understanding and develop greater empathy for others.

Martinez is a Naturopathic Doctor, Occupational Therapist, and Investor. He also enjoys writing, publishing, traveling, blogging AttaBoyCowboy.com, and running his YouTube channel AttaBoyCowboy.

So be sure to check out his fun books, blog, and YouTube channel.

Martinez's work as a Naturopathic Doctor specializes in anti-aging medicine and complementary cancer therapies. He focuses on a whole-body treatment approach utilizing safe natural methods, while simultaneously restoring the body's natural ability to heal.

His work as an Occupational Therapist has allowed him to help people across the lifespan to do things they want and need to do to live their life to the fullest. His strong desire to mentor and help others has led him to teach, share, and help them live better lives.

As an Investor, Martinez has focused his training and business acumen on real estate. With a family history of real estate investing and extensive academic training, he has developed innovative strategies for building wealth from nothing.

In addition to his medical practice and three decades of investing experience, Martinez is making his impact on the writing and media field. Through his books, blog, and YouTube channel, he is reaching a broad spectrum of people and teaching them how to live healthier and wealthier lives.

Martinez has taught extension courses for the University of San Diego in topics ranging from nutrition and general health to leadership and business. He holds five associate degrees from Cerritos College, a bachelor's degree from the University of Southern California (USC), an MBA in economics and marketing, and a master's degree in healthcare management (MHCM) from California State

University Los Angeles (CSULA), a doctoral degree from Clayton College, and over ten other degrees and advanced certifications in areas including lifestyle redesign and nutrition, alternative nutrition, assistive technology, sensory integration, neuro-developmental treatment, physical agent modalities, lymphedema treatment, and property management. He studied over fifteen years working his entire academic career and for several years attending two graduate schools on two separate campuses at the same time.

He is a huge fan of all sports, reading, and being on the road traveling!

As an entrepreneur, Ernesto is usually problem-solving business issues, writing, and learning to be a better person. He enjoys spending time with his family and friends.

By far one of his favorite activities is practicing his Random Acts of Kindness, where he tries to do three acts of kindness for strangers a day.

Bonus

Top Ten Ways to Decrease Your Environmental Impact During Travel per World Wildlife Fund (WWF)

1. Go on holiday during the off-peak period to prevent overstraining resources; you'll also avoid the crowds.

2. Find out about places before you visit. You may be visiting an environmentally sensitive area, in which case you must take extra care to stay on footpaths and follow signs.

3. Don't travel by air if you can avoid it, because air travel uses up large amounts of jet fuel that releases greenhouse gases.

4. Dispose of any rubbish responsibly; it can be hazardous to wildlife.

5. Use public transportation, cycle or walk instead of using a car.

6. Use facilities and trips run by local people whenever possible.

7. Don't be tempted to touch wildlife and disturb habitats whether on land, at the coast, or under water.

8. Be careful what you choose to bring home as a holiday souvenir. Many species from coral and conch shells to elephants and alligators are endangered because they are killed for curios or souvenirs.

9. Don't dump chemicals into the environment; it can be very dangerous for wildlife.

10. Boats and jet-skis create noise and chemical pollution that is very disturbing to wildlife; don't keep the engine running unnecessarily

Top Ten Ways to Decrease Your Environmental Impact after Travel per WWF

1. Completely turn off equipment like televisions and stereos when you're not using them.

2. Choose energy-efficient appliances and light bulbs.

3. Save water: some simple steps can go a long way in saving water, like turning off the tap when you are brushing your teeth or shaving. Try to collect the water used to wash vegetables and salad to water your houseplants.

4. Lower your shades or close your curtains on hot days, to keep the house fresh and reduce the use of electric fans or air-conditioning.

5. Let clothes dry naturally.

6. Keep lids on pans when cooking to conserve energy.

7. Use rechargeable batteries.

8. Call your local government to see if they have a disposal location for used batteries, glass, plastics, paper, or other wastes.

9. Don't use "throwaway" products like paper plates and napkins or plastic knives, forks, and cups.

10. Send electronic greetings over email instead of paper cards.

Top Ten Ways to Decrease Your Environmental Impact in the Garden per WWF

1. Collect rainwater to water your garden.

2. Water the garden early in the morning or late in the evening. Water loss is reduced due to evaporation. Don't over-water the garden. Water only until the soil

becomes moist, not soggy.

3. Explore water-efficient irrigation systems. Sprinkler irrigation and drip irrigation can be adapted to garden situations.

4. Make your garden lively, plant trees, and shrubs that will attract birds. You can also put up bird nest boxes with food.

5. Put waste to work in your garden, sweep the fallen leaves and flowers into flowerbeds, or under shrubs. Increasing soil fertility and also reduce the need for frequent watering.

6. If you have little space in your garden, you could make a compost pit to turn organic waste from the kitchen and garden to soil-enriching manure.

7. Plant local species of trees, flowers, and vegetables.

8. Don't use chemicals in the garden, as they will eventually end up in the water systems and can upset the delicate balance of life cycles.

9. Organic and environmentally friendly fertilizers and pesticides are available - organic gardening reduces pollution and is better for wildlife.

10. Buy fruit and vegetables that are in season to help reduce enormous transport costs resulting from importing products and, where possible, choose locally produced food.

Top Ten Ways to Reduce, Reuse, and Recycle per WWF

1. Use email to stay in touch, including cards, rather than faxing or writing.

2. Share magazines with friends and pass them on to the doctor, dentist, or local hospital for their waiting

rooms.

3. Use recyclable paper to make invitation cards, envelopes, letter pads, etc. if you can.

4. Use washable nappies instead of disposables, if you can.

5. Recycle as much as you can.

6. Give unwanted clothes, toys, and books to charities and orphanages.

7. Store food and other products in containers rather than foil and plastic wrap.

8. When buying fish, look out for a variety of non-endangered species, and buy local fish if possible.

9. Bring your bags to the grocery and refuse plastic bags that create so much waste.

10. Look for products that have less packaging.

Top Ten Ways to Reduce Your Environmental Impact at Work per WWF

1. Always use both sides of a sheet of paper.

2. Use printers that can print on both sides of the paper; try to look into this option when replacing old printers.

3. Use the back of a draft or unwanted printout instead of notebooks. Even with a double-sided printer, there is likely to be plenty of spare paper to use!

4. Always ask for and buy recycled paper if you can, for your business stationery, and to use it in your printers.

5. Switch off computer monitors, printers, and other equipment at the end of each day. Always turn off

your office light and computer monitor when you go out for lunch or to a meeting.

6. Look for power-saving alternatives like LED light bulbs, motion-sensing to control the lighting, LED computer monitors, etc. Prioritize buying or replacing equipment and appliances with their higher Energy Rating alternatives.

7. Contact your energy provider and what they offer in the way of green energy alternatives. You could install solar panels to reduce reliance on energy providers if they're slow on the green energy uptake.

8. Carpool. Ask your workmates that live nearby if they'd be happy to share rides with you.

9. Be smarter with your company vehicles. When reviewing your fleet, spend some time researching more efficient cars.

10. Clean and maintain equipment regularly to extend their useful life and avoid having to replace them. Just like getting your vehicle serviced regularly, your floors, kitchens, equipment, and bathrooms all need regular attention to protect their form and function.

Made in the USA
Coppell, TX
21 August 2021

60904557R10128